A Year Lost and Found

A Year Lost and Found

MICHAEL MAYNE

Foreword by Gerald Priestland

DARTON · LONGMAN + TODD

First published in 1987 by
Darton, Longman and Todd Ltd
1 Spencer Court
140–142 Wandsworth High Street
London SW18 4JJ

Reprinted 2004 (8th printing)

British Library Cataloguing in Publication Data

Mayne, Michael
   A year lost and found.
   1. Sick—Religious life
   I. Title
   248.4   BV4910

   ISBN 0–232–51747–9

Phototypeset by Intype, London
Printed and bound in Great Britain by
Page Bros, Norwich

For the people of Great St Mary's, Cambridge,
and for Alison,
with my love

Foreword

Every author thinks you should read his book; so perhaps
it is as well for him to recruit a second opinion. Being in
that capacity I ought, in turn, to declare my own interests
which are twofold. Michael Mayne was once my boss in
the Religious Department of BBC Radio, so I know very
well the blend of perfectionism and pastoral caring which
shine through these pages. I also have direct experience
of the kind of corrosive infection to which he fell prey.
A close member of my own family started to exhibit
repeated symptoms of heart-attack – alarming at each
occurrence but actually not damaging in their effect – and
it was not until Dr G or H came along that the trouble
was traced to a rare American virus which eventually
burnt itself out leaving no trace. I might hold forth about
the importance of patients harassing their doctors until
they get satisfaction, but that is not Michael's purpose
and I won't exploit the opportunity to dwell on it here.

An old teacher of mine used to insist repeatedly that
'No experience is ever wasted', and that, I believe, is the
message of this book. A crucial year of Michael's life was
lost – and yet he found in it a vein of the purest spiritual
gold. If I may say so, anyone who knew him in the past
was aware that he was intimate with suffering. But now
he takes us with him through a kind of crucifixion and

descent into Hell, up towards resurrection. He would, I am certain, deplore the Christ-like parallel I am hinting at. He would insist that thousands upon thousands of men and women are undergoing worse torments than he. But it is the very ordinariness of the experience that makes his use of it so valuable: here is an apparently cushy cleric at the heart of the ecclesiastical establishment who can speak to us of suffering from what he knows, not from what his theological college taught him. The central insight lies in the words: 'I knew that what I wanted most of all was not to be healed physically, but to learn the lessons of my sickness. I wanted this lost year to be redeemed, to be a valued part of my journey.' And Michael then reminds us that even the Risen Christ still bore the marks of the nails and the spear-wound in his side. The suffering is real, but it is not a dead end.

There is no hero in this book other than the Holy Lord himself; but I hope the perceptive reader will identify three parties who deserve much credit – Michael's wife Alison, the lay leadership of Great St Mary's, and whoever it was at 10 Downing Street who maintained confidence in Michael when some, at least, must have been suggesting a fitter man for the Deanery of Westminster. I think we are all in their debt.

GERALD PRIESTLAND

I greet him the days I meet him, and bless when I understand.

(Gerald Manley Hopkins)[1]

I feel . . . that the world is being made right in front of us, and we stand always at the edge of this creation, and in living out our lives give back piece by piece what has been given to us to use and work and wrestle with. We shape our own lives and find our own humanity in the long passage from premonitions of innocence through the darkness of mortal distress, carelessness and apparent absurdity into the light that we know is there if we have the patience and the courage to be still, to concentrate – to be alert . . .

All is well. Not by facile optimism, not in blinkered evasions, but in the richest and most active dimension of our humanity. It is the illumination we must and will ever seek on the other side of the dark.

(Dennis Potter)[2]

Preface

This is not a theological book about healing. The awesome mystery of the human body, and how matter is wedded to spirit, is something which as yet I understand only a little.

Nor is it a book about prayer in times of sickness. I have learned I am not very good at that.

It is unashamedly a very personal book about one year of my life, and what a sudden, mysterious knock-down kind of illness does to you and your family; about doctors and their still limited knowledge in certain areas; and about a God who stops you dead in your tracks and sets you groping for answers.

I do not claim to have found the answers, just 'hints and guesses'; nor as yet to have learned many lessons, but I think I begin to understand how all this apparent waste and frustration can make sense as part of my own inner journey.

When it comes to revealing your inner self, insofar as you know it, there is an understandable reticence, a natural and often proper reserve. (I can already hear certain friends saying of what follows: 'A useful bit of therapy for himself, no doubt, but better left unpublished.') And yet such a reluctance to share our small experience of God and our deepest convictions about him

1

in a personal and vulnerable way is reflected in whole libraries of sound but dead theology, and can be heard in a thousand distanced, objective sermons. It is not that the words are untrue, but somehow they fail to be earthed.

Sometimes speakers at the term-time evening university service at Great St Mary's, Cambridge, would ask for advice. The only advice I have ever wanted to give is this: 'If it is in your nature to do so, be a little vulnerable. Don't be afraid to talk about yourself, *your* journey, *your* pain, *your* vision.' And some of the most memorable speakers have done so.

I do not believe this kind of speaking about ourselves need be self-indulgent, though one of the worst things about illness is how self-centred we can become, how our days (and more especially the nights) centre on symptoms and states of feeling, and every new pain is ominous.

But I do believe that all human beings, unique and different in so many respects, share the more profound experience of love and grief, joy and suffering, and can afford to be more open and honest with each other. There is an entry in Philip Toynbee's diary (*Part of a Journey*) to this effect:

15.3.79. We had to go and have drinks with a couple . . . [He] was a sporting businessman, and as we were talking I realised that there were three possible levels of communication between him and me:
a. our present one, making polite, meaningless noises to each other;
b. the angry argument which would certainly follow if we stumbled into any social or political issue;
c. the confession that we are fellow men, full of fear and anguish, calling for help.
(a) and (b) are not really communication at all; but

2

how seldom, even with old friends, do we ever communicate on the third level. Yet it is only there, in the sharing of affliction and helplessness, that the fruit of love can grow.[3]

What follows is an honest attempt to communicate 'on the third level', to describe what it has been like, as a busy parish priest, to find I am not indispensable, trying to trust that God is there with me, deep in the heart of it. And, indeed, that he has a very strange sense of timing which he alone understands.

I have written as a layman in medical matters and deliberately not sought any medical expertise which was not offered at the time. For what follows is not intended to convey what has been actually happening to me in this 'undiagnosed viral infection', but what it has felt like.

The book is in two parts, with a postscript. The first part, from May 1985 to April 1986, is a record of those months. The second part, headed May 1986, is a reflection upon them. In it I have tried to describe how illness affected my family life and my understanding of priesthood. And I have tried to ask large questions about such mysteries as the meaning of the Cross, suffering and redemption.

The greater part of this small book was written in a village high in the Dolomites, in what is their spring. I began it in the days leading up to Pentecost and finished it on the Wednesday in Whit week. For once I was not surrounded by books containing other people's words and ideas, but by mountains still covered by snow, with the first gentians and pasque flowers appearing in the silent woods and the meadows carpeted with oxlip and tiny white and purple crocus.

It had been exactly a year . . .

Part I

It was the day of the Heysel football match, and as I drove home from a private retreat the fields of rape and the new corn glinting in the evening sun were in grim contrast to the horror of the unfolding toll of deaths on the car radio. Those who had been due to comment on the match were moved almost to tears by the violence on the terraces. I had been with a small community of nuns at Peakirk, near the birthplace of the poet John Clare at Helpston, and between saying the offices and times of reading and prayer, I walked the country paths known and celebrated in prose and verse by that sad and lovely man.

But increasingly I felt unwell, strangely inert, with swollen glands, discomfort in the neck and shoulders and mild pains in the chest. I put it down to the general malaise of middle age. After all, I was in my mid-fifties, and six years at Great St Mary's had taken their toll. It is a demanding place: a lot of administration, much pastoral counselling, and the expectation that a constant stream of well-known, interesting speakers – churchmen, politicians, artists, scientists – will come and speak each

5

Sunday night of term, with all the detailed correspon-
dence and planning that involves.

In February there had taken place 'Encounters', an
ecumenical teaching week led by the Archbishop of
Canterbury, supported by (among others) Archbishop
Derek Worlock, Bishop David Sheppard, Colin Morris,
Una Kroll, Myra Blyth, Rowan Williams and Jack Domi-
nian. It was the outcome of two years' work by a
committee of deans and chaplains and students which I
had chaired. Hard on its heels came Lent and Holy Week,
and a few days' watching birds on the Norfolk coast had
not done much to restore my energy.

In addition I was desperately trying to find time to write
a series of priests' ordination addresses for the Diocese
of Chelmsford in the middle of June. Their theme? The
need for a priest to have a stillness and a space at the
centre of his being, with time to observe the natural
world; a love for people; the understanding of the nature
of forgiveness; and an ability to give thanks 'at all times
and in all places': in a word, what it means to live euchar-
istically. At one level I was aware, not of hypocrisy for I
deeply believed what I was saying, but of a dangerous
echo of Parson Williams, Rector of Llanbedr a hundred
years ago, of whom Kilvert wrote in his diaries that he
would thump his pulpit and say to his people, 'My
brethren, don't you do as I *do*, but you do as I *say*!'

June

But the Lord had other things in mind.

I battled with the addresses, and for refreshment went
on the last Sunday night of term to the Madrigals, sung

by the University Chamber Choir from punts moored to the river bank. At dusk there is a magical moment when the coloured lights are lit and the punts drift down the Cam. Not for me: the whole of the left side of my neck was swollen as if with mumps and I felt drained and thoroughly miserable.

Two days later, I took my daughter Sarah to the Footlights and sat there speculating on what might be wrong with me and imagining the worst. On the following day there was the annual evening barbecue for some sixty students in our garden, those who had contributed to Great St Mary's by acting as sidesmen, readers, servers or college representatives. In the afternoon I cycled to say farewell to an elderly couple about to move away from Cambridge. It was to be the last pastoral visit for quite a while. Half-way through tea my arms and legs felt that they had turned to lead, and trying to cycle home was like cycling through sand. I gave up and went to bed, with the smell of hamburgers being barbecued beneath the window.

A week later Hans Küng was to receive an honorary degree, and we were invited to dine with him the previous evening. Foolishly I went, boringly explaining to my somewhat surprised fellow guests that I needed to sit down all the time and that they must forgive me if I didn't talk very much.

That Sunday I preached. It left me exhausted – and where had my voice gone? It was strangely diminished and it made my lungs ache to talk. On the Tuesday I walked a few hundred yards to a meeting of a committee seeking to establish a centre for the meths drinkers and permanently unemployed, but when I tried to walk back the few hundred yards to the church I collapsed conveniently on the doorstep of the Cyrenians' Hostel for the Homeless and had to be revived with strong tea.

Stubborn to the end, two days later I insisted on going to Pleshey for the ordination retreat. All the addresses were written, and a combination of responsibility and pride made me think I could still deliver them. Luckily my wife Alison came with me, knowing different. The first address hardly reached the first row of the small chapel: my whole power of projection had gone, and feeling light-headed and rather foolish, I was ordered to leave by the bishop and driven home.

My GP, who had already seen me twice and told me to go slow, is a man of extreme gentleness and reticence. An admirable, listening doctor, he is reluctant to diagnose and tends to leave many decisions to his patients. I like him immensely, and our friendship has survived a year of frequent visits to the surgery, where much of the time the most he could offer was encouragement and the belief that in the end all would be well. At that stage, he gave me a complete overhaul, took various blood tests, and said he thought he could hear a bit of 'creaking' in my right lung. He arranged for me to have an X-ray and promised to report back on the blood tests.

A week later, one of the tests showed a slightly high toxoplasmic level, and the likelihood was that I had toxoplasmosis, an enervating blood disease which takes a good while to clear. I was referred to a specialist in blood diseases, Dr A, and told that he could not see me for three weeks. In the meantime I sat in discomfort and weakness and waited. On good days it was a real achievement to walk once, very slowly, round our modest garden.

July

Wimbledon and, a little later, the Australian Test series came and went. They provided some small diversion at an otherwise bleak time: days which fell into a predictable pattern through a mercifully cool summer, in which the high spots became a Guinness before lunch, and sometimes a carefully selected visitor at teatime. Once round the garden was still the daily norm. One moonlit evening I unwisely went round four times and paid for it for several days. It sounds absurd, but that's how it was.

When people asked 'How are you?' during this long summer and autumn it was hard to gauge how much they really wanted to know. I was only too ready to enlarge on what had become so important a subject: 'I feel as weak as a kitten. My arms ache constantly. My chest feels bruised and at night I cannot lie on either side without the probability of being woken by pain. But the most tedious thing' (and by now eyes had begun to glaze a little, smiles to become fixed) 'is that I can't sit comfortably in my chair. My glands in the neck and chest around the thorax are so swollen that I have to sit upright, and the slightest pressure on my back makes me feel ill. And, for good measure, my brain is not working awfully well; I forget things and find it hard to concentrate.'

But really it was better to say little or nothing, hard as that was, for one of the dispiriting things about any long illness is that you become so boring, driven in upon yourself, your world contracted to four walls upstairs, four walls down.

On 19th July I saw Doctor A, or rather his Registrar. The latter gave me a complete overhaul and reassured me that the toxoplasmosis (which seemed the likeliest

9

diagnosis) would pass in time, though I should allow about five months for safety. Doctor A then appeared and encouraged me to keep a planned holiday in September. He asked for the X-ray: it was not to be found, so I was sent off to have another. 'I'll have the result next Thursday,' he said. 'Come and see me on my ward round.'

The following week I sat with Alison in the visitors' waiting room. Doctor A appeared, holding both X-rays. The first showed a white patch on the lung – fluid, apparently – while the second seemed more or less normal. 'Nothing to worry about there', he said as he flourished them, 'A touch of viral pneumonia, but the infection seems to have cleared up.'

'But I can hardly walk fifty yards,' I replied. 'How long will it be before I recover?'

He was very properly guarded, and went on to explain that it depended on my immune system and how it responds. 'It could be a fortnight, or a month; it could be three months – even six.' He invited me to come back on 2nd September.

August

During August the pains in the chest got worse: short bouts like severe indigestion, and a kind of gnawing discomfort in the lung area. A phone call came from my GP: 'The final blood tests have come back. It *isn't* toxoplasmosis – that was a past infection.'

So what was it?

'It seems to be a viral infection of some kind – undiagnosed as yet – not unlike glandular fever. I'm a bit concerned about the pains in your chest. Would you like

10

to see Doctor B as well as Doctor A? He's a heart-and-lungs man.'

'How soon can it be arranged?'

'Pretty soon, I guess.'

I saw Doctor B on the 10th, after further X-rays. I liked him at once. Almost his first question was, 'Tell me what it *feels* like'. He was puzzled by the X-rays. There was something not quite right, though he couldn't put his finger on it. He gave me lots of time (which explained the endless waiting in his clinic corridors), then arranged for further blood tests and breathing tests, the sort where you blow into tubes which analyse the proportion of oxygen and hydrogen your lungs are receiving. He arranged to see me when I was also due to see Doctor A on 2nd September.

'People at Great St Mary's are finding it hard to adjust to a nameless illness. So am I. What shall I call it?'

'Tell them it's pleurisy; it's as good a name as any other.'

August followed the pattern of July, and September and October. I listened to music, a lot of Mozart and Bach and Verdi, and those haunting settings of Blake's poems by Vaughan Williams; and read as much as I could, mainly novels and a bit of poetry, Yeats and R. S. Thomas. I couldn't cope with theology, with two exceptions: Angela Tilby's *Won't You Join the Dance?* and Tony Bridge's *One Man's Advent*. They passed my tests for humanity and vulnerability as well as being imaginative attempts to answer the questions people actually ask about God. I did a few large jigsaws, and felt unreasonable rage if bits were missing.

But for quite a lot of the time I sat and observed. I had normally written a monthly parish Newsletter, on a whole range of subjects from the morality of nuclear deterrence to test-tube babies or the nature of the Resurrection. They rarely got any response. For the September letter I wrote this, and called it 'Watching the Beans Grow'.

For three months my world has consisted of a room with a radio, books and a view of the garden, and it seems likely to do so for a few weeks longer. Lots of music, some good novels, wondering if Guinness and Lucozade really *are* good for you, being for once at the receiving end,
  '. . . cabined, cribbed, confined, bound in
  To saucy doubts and fears.'
'At least it will give you time to pray,' wrote a friend. But no; when you are ill you need others within the Body to do that for you.
  Instead I have watched my beans grow, rocked by the wind, rejoicing in the scarlet flowers and the fast-growing pods, unleashing my anger on the blackfly; and seen how the few last leeks, deliberately undug, have gone to seed, the heads first swelling, then the paper-thin cover breaking and the spectacular spiky flower gradually turning a shade of lilac.
  I know at what time the spotted fly-catchers will appear, perch on the cherry tree and begin their darting flight over the lawn; and where the pair of goldfinch has been nesting; and on the rare fine evening I have watched the evening light as it spreads across the garden and clothes a single rose with a kind of glory.
  Am I about to draw a conclusion, point a moral in good Thought for the Day fashion? No, not this time. I leave that to you. And send my love.

To my surprise people wrote to me about it. I had been half ashamed of its Patience Strong overtones but it seemed to touch a nerve. No doubt some were glad that

I had been forced to slow down and in one particular way begin to practise what I preached.

One question I had to face during these passive, uncomfortable months was what form my prayer life should take. While not obsessive about the saying of the offices of morning and evening prayer, my practice was to say them with others daily in the chapel at Great St Mary's, and to celebrate or participate in the Eucharist on most weekdays. Now I was brought Communion once a week at home, but I had neither the will nor the desire to say the offices. After a bit, I compromised and said a form of truncated morning prayer which largely consisted of the Jubilate and the psalm of the day, and (if I felt like it) a bit of the New Testament. I had always known with my mind that the Psalms are an incomparable storehouse of wisdom and strength: now I discovered in my heart that time and again they spoke astonishingly to my very condition of desolation and despair, and could reassure me of the love and presence of God. A phrase would leap from the page and lift my heart.

There are the cries for help:

My God, I cry to you but you do not answer,
and by night also I take no rest . . .[4]

Why do you stand so far off, O Lord?
why do you hide your face in time of need?[5]

How long must I suffer anguish in my soul
and be so grieved in my heart day and night?[6]

The waves of death encompassed me,
and the floods of chaos overwhelmed me . . .

In my anguish I called to the Lord,
I cried for help from my God.[7]

13

But as well as the cries for help there are the cries of thanksgiving for reassurance. So that within the same psalms we find:

Why are you so full of heaviness my soul:
   and why so unquiet within me?
O put your trust in God:
   for I will praise him yet
   who is my deliverer and my God.[8]

Thou art about my path and about my bed . . .
   When I wake up I am present with thee.[9]

If I say, 'Surely the darkness will cover me:
   and the night will enclose me,'
the darkness is no darkness with you
but the night is as clear as the day:
   the darkness and the light are both alike.[10]

Heaviness may endure for a night
   but joy comes in the morning.[11]

Even so, there were a few times during these dragging summer months, when every morning brought a difficult day and every evening a more difficult night (thank God for sleeping pills!), and when the very frustration of not getting better reduced me to tears, tears not of rage or anger – or not often – but just, I suppose, of plain self-pity. Mercifully I was at no time clinically depressed, just diminished and frustrated. I need to say more about our understanding of God which can be part of the healing process, and which may be the one thing one can hold on to in times of weakness and sickness; but a little later.

Visitors were sometimes a problem; however sensitive, they were always tiring. But on the whole those who knew what was required of a visitor of the sick came, and those who thought discretion was the better part of sick-visiting sent cards and messages. But what interested me was what people did when they came, especially my fellow priests. 'As sickness is the greatest misery', wrote John Donne, 'so the great misery of sickness is solitude . . . solitude is a torment which is not threatened in Hell itself.'[12] You *do* feel cut off, and you do need reassuring. And the best and most effective way of achieving both is by touch and by prayer. I was so grateful to the small number of priests who overcame their understandable shyness with a fellow-priest and laid hands on me and blessed me; and I knew which way I should decide in future when visiting sick people either at home or in hospital. Often I have been undecided as to what is needed: a prayer, a blessing – with or without the laying-on of hands; or neither. Now I know; and if I err it will be because I believe that most of us, when we are sick, need physical contact and the spoken assurance of God's love. Other things as well, of course (books and grapes and gossip), but those most of all.

Any conversation – using the lungs – remained exhausting, but I achieved one creative thing: I spent an hour each morning editing *Encounters* (Darton, Longman and Todd, 1986).

September

On the 2nd of September, walking at a geriatric pace and stopping often in the endless hospital corridors, I discovered Doctor A was away and saw yet another Registrar. I had the usual general overhaul: blood pressure, pulse, liver, lungs, and all seemed fine. He passed me on to the X-ray unit for a further X-ray, followed by another session with Doctor B. The blood tests were pretty normal, and he was confident it must be a viral infection, but still finding the X-rays a little puzzling he suggested an appointment in a week's time at a different hospital for an electrocardiagram and further breathing tests.

They revealed nothing abnormal. The ECG, in which pads are attached to your body and your heart is monitored while you walk on a treadmill whose pace is increasing each minute, was a shock after the gentle stroll round the garden, and after four minutes I buckled at the knees.

A week later I panicked. The chest pains had severely increased, and I would wake in the small hours, my neck-pulse pounding, with a sense that a great weight was crushing my lungs. Doctor B was now on holiday, but his Registrar saw me at once and had me X-rayed yet again. He took great care, and to my somewhat indignant relief, reassured me that nothing appeared to be organically wrong. It seemed to me at that moment that it would have been so much easier if something had been. Of course that's nonsense: it would have been far worse. It is just that people understand a well-labelled disease like a tumour or a heart attack and can relate to it. As it was, few were familiar with an illness so hard to diagnose, and they were puzzled that I was not visibly improving, but rather the reverse. Helpful messages would suggest that a friend of a friend 'had just what you've got and woke up one morning feeling quite well again'. (And the less helpful had friends of friends whose symptoms lasted for years.)

M understood. A physician himself, he had a similar virus which lasted five months and from which he had fully recovered. He came to see me and reassured me by

16

the very fact that he knew what it was like, but warned me that it could take a good many more months to play itself out. Luckily I did not know at the time just how many.

I now felt that if the doctors could do no more than tell me to wait in patience, then perhaps someone from the world of alternative medicine would help. I wasn't short of advice, nor is Cambridge short of such practitioners. A friend advised acupuncture, and in particular a Vietnamese doctor who practised it. I went on 20th September to her small council house. Thinking about it now, there wasn't a dog's chance of it working. From childhood I have had a phobia about needles and often pass out at the first whiff of an injection. It was crazy, but in September I was ready to pin my hopes on anything.

Doctor C was slim and charming and wholly understood my hang-up. We had a gentle introductory session. She placed a discreet needle or two at the acupuncture points, chiefly in the chest and feet. I could not have been more calm. We booked a second session within days. This time, though, it was for real: needles in my back, chest, feet, and – final horror – a tiny needle implanted in my ear with instructions to keep it in for a week. I became obsessed with that needle, especially as I had been encouraged to press it gently when I felt short of energy, which was most of the time. I pulled it out in the middle of the night and decided that the ancient and therapeutic art of acupuncture was not for me.

I wasn't sure what to try next. I thought of the Emperor Menelik II, the dynamic and resourceful creator of modern Ethiopia, who was in the habit of nibbling a few pages of the Bible whenever he became ill. In December 1913, while recovering from a stroke, he ate the entire Book of Kings and died.

Some suggested healing of a more specifically Christian kind. For example, I was given the names of two individuals with undoubted gifts of healing. One lived in Cheshire; the other, more local, man was strongly charismatic. Rightly or wrongly, I decided against seeing him. It is not that I doubt the reality of the charismatic renewal and its transforming effect on some who have found liberation at an emotional level and healing of a physical kind. But something deep in me mistrusts many of its manifestations, and however much I might be groping for help, I knew it had to be help from God working through agents with whom I was basically sympathetic and whom I could wholly trust.

I think now, although I was unaware of it at the time, that my instinctive resistance to any kind of 'immediate' charismatic healing was because of my deeply ingrained belief that God would heal me quietly and unobtrusively through the natural – but no less miraculous – power of my body to renew itself, what you might call its inbuilt instinct for life and health. The God who creates and re-creates is constantly at work. What matters is that we recognise that fact and co-operate with, and are open to, God's creative life within us.

And there was no doubt that God's love was being mediated to me in a number of ways. Certainly I was not short of prayer, fully aware of the support of the community at Great St Mary's and others outside it. In addition, during all this time, my weekly Communion was sometimes brought by Leslie Brown, a wise and good friend, one-time Archbishop in Uganda, now retired and increasingly blind. He insisted on walking the mile from town to the vicarage, crossing main roads with calm but unwise abandon, and he brought his own quiet and authoritative presence to the house. Always he laid hands on

18

me, and on occasion he anointed me; and it distressed me always to have to report that I seemed little better. That is not to say that God's healing power was not at work through him, just that I longed to feel some change in myself and didn't. I think now I know why.

October

I had a target: Princess Anne was coming on 13th October to speak at the University service about the Save the Children Fund. Although I couldn't put questions to her as planned, I was determined to be there, at least to welcome and introduce her. And so I was, though my chest felt heavy and I ached for days afterwards; and Princess Anne was superb, a persuasive protagonist for the needs of the Third World, really listening to questions from students and others in the congregation and dodging nothing.

Having seen me in public some people assumed I was well again. That was an indication of problems to come: how you ease yourself infinitely slowly back into the life of the community, without raising expectations you cannot hope to meet. 'How are you?' – never the easiest of questions to answer – soon becomes by implication, at least in the sick person's ears, 'Why are you not better?'

Three days later I went, at Doctor B's suggestion, for a lung scan. You lie still on the great machine for forty minutes while it reads off your lungs inch by inch. A week later I saw Doctor B. The lungs were fine. He took time to explain what he called the 'post-viral syndrome', a kind of depression of the body – not of the mind – where what is known as the circadian rhythm has been disrupted and needs restoring; not unlike permanent jet-lag. He recommended (at last!) a course of pills.

'What will they do?'

'Help restore your circadian rhythm. They have proved very effective with rats.'

'What are they?'

'Anti-depressants.'

'But I'm not depressed.'

Doctor B sighed, but in a kindly way. I hadn't been listening. That was the trouble: it was so hard to concentrate. He signed me off and passed me back to Doctor A.

I took the pills home, swallowed the first dose, and then perversely but following some deep instinct, threw the lot away.

Those who had been seeing us most frequently now began making encouraging noises about getting a change of air. Certainly Alison, who had borne the brunt of it and had been for a while deeply anxious, needed a break. We agreed to go for a week to Hengrave Hall, an ecumenical centre set in a beautiful manor house in Suffolk. Those in charge were kindness itself, but the combination of corridors and stairs (stop at every fifth stair) and the need to make conversation, added to the constant need to try to explain what was wrong, showed me how physically and spiritually weak I still was, quite unable to cope. We came home the following day.

At that low point, with nothing in view before a further appointment with Doctor A on 9th December, I kept on hearing of a retired surgeon, an old man of eighty, who now practised as a holistic doctor. As soon as I met Doctor D, I recognised a man of wide experience, wisdom and spirituality. We met as persons: he was concerned with me as an embodied spirit, and with the power of God which could be set free to restore me.

But he was also concerned with the nuts and bolts; with the three great keys to health: breathing, posture and diet. He tested the level of my natural and psychic energy and found it to be nil. He manipulated my limbs and found them to have all the stiffness of those of 'the public man', the professional who must in some sense perform in public. He gave me breathing exercises and told me what I instinctively knew but needed to learn again, how to relax and find physical and mental stillness.

Then he 'doused' me, though he had a more professional word for it himself. I lay on a table stripped to the waist, my left arm at forty-five degrees to my body. He placed his hand over mine, exerting sufficient pressure for me to keep the arm raised with a small effort. Then, one by one, he placed some three dozen small medicine bottles containing a different ingredient on my solar plexus. My hand either held the tension with his and remained firm; or at once dropped. The bottles which caused the first reaction went in one bowl: those which caused my arm to drop went in the other. He then made me list those foodstuffs which I had better avoid if my system was to have the best chance of regaining its strength: coffee, cheese, eggs, tomatoes, teabags, pasta, white flour, gluten, yeast, beef, lamb – the list seemed endless.

'For how long?'

'Until you are better.'

'And then can I eat normally again?'

'Yes, though if you are wise you will not drink coffee again.'

'Never?'

'Never.'

21

No mention was made of alcohol and I didn't ask.

The diet was harder on Alison than on me, but she did wonders with fish and chicken, fruit and salad. At the same time I was taking some homeopathic pills, together with the only thing that twice a day brought some relief: a mild muscle relaxant. For part of the trouble now was muscular as well as glandular. Until May I had cycled everywhere, always moved quickly, run upstairs, used my hands a lot in talking. Now for months I had moved from one chair to another and everything had seized up. Doctor D tried to get me going again, and I paid half a dozen visits to him over the next few months. He talked and he tested or massaged parts of my body. Sometimes he just talked. He had the great gift of encouragement. He understood that the question 'How are you?' is at root a metaphysical question, which is not sufficiently answered with clinical lists and data (blood pressure, pulse rate, urinalysis and so on), but goes to the deepest part of ourselves as the complex and uniquely precious beings we are.

(A month after I had written these words, Doctor D died peacefully after a sudden heart attack. He was a good man who had given his life to healing in the widest sense.)

At about the same time I read two books by the remarkable British neurologist, Oliver Sacks, who has worked for many years at a large hospital in the United States which he calls 'Mount Carmel'. The first book, *Awakenings*, deals with the discovery of the drug L-DOPA, and its often frighteningly dramatic effect on Parkinsonian patients suffering from the disease *encephalitis lethargica*, sometimes known as 'sleeping sickness'. The second book, *A Leg to Stand On*, is about a serious accident Sacks suffered while climbing in Norway, when his leg

22

was wrenched from its socket and the main tendon ruptured, and his astonished discovery of the delusions and frustrations a normally sane and rational person can undergo in hospital, and what it is like to have the roles reversed and to be a patient. Both books (recently published in paperback) have profound things to say about healing and what it means properly to treat a person who is sick.

Sacks writes of the dialogue necessary between patient and doctor which can only be held 'if there is a direct and human confrontation, an "I–Thou" relation . . .' He goes on:

> There is nothing alive which is not individual: our health is *ours*; our diseases are *ours*; our reactions are *ours* – no less than our minds or our faces. Our health, diseases, and reaction cannot be understood *in vitro*, in themselves; they can only be understood with reference to *us*, as expressions of our nature, our living, our being-here in the world. Yet modern medicine, increasingly, dismisses our existence, either reducing us to identical replicas reacting to fixed 'stimuli' in equally fixed ways, or seeing our diseases as purely alien and bad, without organic relation to the person who is ill . . . Diseases have a character of their own, but they also partake of our character; we have a character of our own, but we also partake of the world's character . . . the disease—the man—the world go together, and cannot be considered separately as things-in-themselves . . .[13]

We are never simply concerned with a handful of 'symptoms', but with a *person* and his changing relation to the world. Moreover, the language we need must be both particular and general, combining reverence to the patient and *his* nature, and to the world and *its* nature.[14]

Sacks describes in detail, in *Awakenings*, the case-history of individual patients who are treated with L-DOPA. Many have been, for as long as fifty years, in a state as good as dead, conscious of their surroundings but motionless and speechless, confined to asylums or other institutions. When the drug was given many experienced a kind of resurrection, though their reaction was varied and unpredictable. Some maintained this new life and functioned with a high degree of normality; others regressed. Why? Always it depended on there being one person – a relative, a friend – to love them and give them value. Those who are alone in the world (Donne's 'state of solitude') regress: those who are loved find at least a degree of healing they would not otherwise have known.

In dealing with deeply ill patients, a prerequisite is the establishment of proper relations with the world, and – in particular – with other human beings, or *one* human being, for it is human relations which carry the possibilities of proper being-in-the-world. Feeling the fullness of the presence of the world depends on feeling the fullness of another *person*, as a person; reality is given to us by the reality of people; our sense of reality, of trust or security, is critically dependent on a human relation. A single good relation is a lifeline . . . and we see, again and again in the histories of these patients, how a single relation can extricate them from trouble. Kinship is healing; we are physicians to each other.[15]

Finally, speaking of the place of hospitals such as Mount Carmel for long-term or terminal patients, Sacks concludes:

24

The essential function of such hospitals – which house several millions of the world's population – is that they shall provide *hospitality*, the feeling of home, for patients who have lost their original homes. To the extent that Mount Carmel acts as a *home* it is deeply therapeutic to all of its patients; to the extent that it acts as an *institution*, it deprives them of their sense of reality and home, and forces them into the false-homes and compensations of regression and sickness . . . The work of healing, of rendering whole, is, first and last, the business of love.[16]

November

By now the most draining weakness had passed, and each day I would walk for about fifteen minutes round Churchill College playing fields, opposite our house. We therefore decided to have another shot at a change of scene. Alison drove by stages to my mother in Devon; then we spent five days at a hotel near Stratford. I found I could walk a little, but any kind of exertion, such as talking too much or walking too far, or going to the Theatre Royal to see a charming *As You Like It*, brought on the old feelings of pain and pressure in the lungs, almost a feeling of suffocation; and any pressure on the back brought a sense of nausea. That, over the months, became the most tiresome and wearing of symptoms. It is such a small thing, I am half ashamed to mention it; yet if this journal of an illness is going to speak to others with similar devastating viruses, who find medical knowledge is still exploring this area, then such tedious accuracy may help.

The symptoms had in fact changed a bit by now: much less weakness in the limbs, less frequent pain in the chest – just nagging discomfort; but the glands in the neck and shoulders were still swollen, and it felt as though I had a permanently stiff neck from the eye to the upper jaw and right down to the breastbone, with a monotonous niggling ache just under the collar-bone.

About this time *The Observer* published a report of a girl with not dissimilar symptoms who turned out to have mercury poisoning from the fillings in her teeth. A few weeks before, a friend visiting South Africa had persuaded me to let her take some strands of my hair to a neighbour in Durban who had strange powers of analysis. She put it in her 'black box' and at once diagnosed mercury poisoning or, less likely, lead poisoning. Open to any suggestion, I went to see my dentist. He was not impressed. 'A very fashionable illness,' he said, with the air of one who knows it's a lot of baloney. But to please me he took some X-rays and they seemed normal enough. So we forgot about that.

But it was in Stratford that the bomb fell. I had asked my son to forward any letters that looked urgent or particularly interesting. On the second morning there was a large envelope from him. Inside was an envelope marked 'Private and confidential'. It was a request for a reference. But, just by chance, Mark had included another envelope which looked a bit formal but said nothing on the outside. Inside, however, a second envelope said 'Strictly private and confidential' and contained a letter from the Prime Minister asking me to let my name go forward for the Deanery of Westminster.

It was a thoughtful and considerate letter, which spoke of my illness, told me there was time for proper consideration, and that much would depend on the reports not only of my own doctors but of the doctor who advises the Government in these matters. Finally and understandably, I was only allowed to speak to a very few close and trusted advisers.

At any time such an invitation would be daunting, though exciting too; and I would have needed time to talk and pray about it in order to make as sure as possible that this thing was of God. But now? I felt so withdrawn from my normal world, so out of touch with my normal instincts and emotions, so bewildered and demoralised by this tedious, undiagnosable thing which had dragged me down for nearly seven months, that the whole proposition seemed unreal, impossible. How could I leave Great St Mary's after doing no work and leading no worship for what might be the best part of a year? How could I cope with a large job with all the new expectations that would bring unless I was fully restored to health? And what guarantee was there of that?

Within a week or two the doctors had been consulted. They replied in the only way they could. There had been no diagnosis, there could be no certain prognosis. Yet the likelihood was that most cases of viral infection clear up in about a year, and my GP suggested that, while I was unlikely to be fit by Easter, the chances that I should be fit by the summer were reasonably good. Certainly there had been progress. Doctor A saw me at the hospital and, in his turn, talked a little about what is known of the 'post-viral muscle fatigue syndrome'. At first, progress would almost certainly be creepingly slow; second, increasingly there would be good periods, followed by setbacks; third, there was a 98 per cent chance that I would fully recover.

Meanwhile I talked with three wise and perceptive people, who know me and Westminster Abbey. They said

I should accept. My own instincts said the same, although at that stage I didn't really trust my own judgement. And so, for once in my life, I trusted the judgement of others and put my faith in the fact that, while God's sense of timing may be strange, he is not a practical joker and will be able in ways quite unknown to me to use me in that place.

December

So, in the third week of December, I wrote back to the Prime Minister and said 'Yes', recognising that everything now depended on the acceptance of the doctors' reports. There followed almost the worst time, for Christmas and the New Year intervened, and it was a good fortnight before I knew I had been appointed and a date for the announcement was agreed: 26th January.

As soon as I knew I might be leaving, I felt it important that I should be seen again in action in my church. I celebrated first on a weekday early in the month, half-chaired a meeting of the parochial church council, and read the gospel at the parish communion for the next two Sundays. But each time I was left feeling weak and exhausted, and wondered afresh at the wisdom of agreeing to go to Westminster Abbey. On the Sunday before Christmas I baptised some babies at the Eucharist, and on Christmas Day I actually celebrated at the parish communion.

The week after Christmas knocked me flat. It was one of Doctor A's 'times of setback' and over the next few months I got to know them well, though it was hard not to feel disappointed and resentful. 'What are you doing to me, God? I long to be well: I put my trust in your healing power: why are you so slow?' I still had a lot to learn.

January 1986

For some months a good friend who has an interest in psychic matters had been encouraging me to contact a woman, Mrs F, who, like the South African who tested my hair, diagnoses at a distance and has remarkable powers of clairvoyance. He had given her my name, no more; and urged me to ring her. Eventually, on a low day in January, I did. She told me she already had several foolscap pages of notes about me, which was a little alarming, and first diagnosed a weakness in the kidneys, then in the liver. This was a new line. She told me my psychic energy was nil, said she would work on it, and that I should expect to feel better. I have no doubt of her strange and unusual powers, nor that she is used by God to help a great many people; but I am slightly uneasy in this borderline world. Nevertheless I phoned her again a fortnight later, to be told that it was undoubtedly my liver, that I had probably picked up the original virus at a funeral when I was physically in a low state of health, and that there was one particular food I needed to eat above all others.

'What is that?'

'I'll tell you in a moment . . . it's just escaping me . . .'

There was a longish pause. 'Oh,' she said in surprise, 'I've never been given that one before. It's duck.'

'*Duck*? But I haven't eaten duck for years.'

'You should, it obviously contains something your body

29

badly needs.' And she added, 'One meal could do the trick'.

An hour later Alison and I went out to supper with an old friend, only the second time we had been out in months. She produced, to our astonishment, roast duck.

'Why did you choose to give us this?'

'It's the *Good Housekeeping* recipe of the month'.

The following day I telephoned Mrs F and told her.

'Oh yes', she said, 'We have to remember that God moves in mysterious ways.'

I've eaten duck twice since then, and each time think of Mrs F with affection, and convince myself it's doing me good.

On 12th January I preached again for the first time, using the story of the eighteenth camel as a recognition that I was dispensable, but also as a warning shot, which only my closest colleagues could appreciate, for what I would have to tell them all two weeks later. The story is of an Arab who had three sons. When he died, he left instructions in his will that his property should be divided up in a certain way. Everything was quite straightforward except for his camels, of which there were seventeen. The will said that half were to go to the eldest son, a third to the middle son, and a ninth to the youngest. How do you divide seventeen camels by two, three or nine, without having bits left over? Finally, in desperation, they went to a neighbour and asked his advice. The neighbour said: 'I have a camel. I will lend it to you and you will find that everything is resolved.' So he did, and once they had eighteen camels it was very simple: the eldest son got a half (nine camels), the second a third (six camels), and the youngest a ninth (two camels), making seventeen camels in all. The neighbour then took his own camel back, and all was well. The story has profound implications for any who are professional counsellors, who may need to be called in to help people sort out their lives at particular moments, or priests who may come to serve a particular community for a limited number of years, but who must not allow others to become so totally dependent upon them that they cannot withdraw when their particular job is done.

The next day my GP suggested, as I was still experiencing a lot of muscular weakness and discomfort, that I should go to Oxford for a session on a nuclear magnetic resonance machine. This is part of a research project to analyse muscular reaction in the 'post-viral fatigue syndrome' and is housed in the old Radcliffe Infirmary. You lie with your arm plunged into a hole and magnetised, rhythmically squeezing a rubber ball with your hand. As I understand it, the computer monitors the acids released by your muscles and tests if things are working as they should. It was an interesting morning, but it failed to prove anything either way, as I was warned might be the case.

By the end of the month I was deliberately doing what I could – though that did not amount to more than assisting at one service each Sunday – in order to reduce the shock of the announcement I had to make at the end of the parish communion on the 26th. These things are always painful on both sides. Afterwards, one natural reaction was 'Thank God, you must be fully well again', and once more it was hard to respond without sounding negative or dishonest. In fact a few days earlier a boy of nineteen had been tragically killed in a car crash, and suddenly I was badly needed by his deeply grieving parents. I arranged the funeral/memorial service and gave the address. I found myself once again speaking of what it means to trust God in the face of such an appalling tragedy, and speaking about the power and love of God who, however long it takes, can bring good out of something which at the time can only seem wholly destructive. That night I began to feel that I had been able to cope again as a priest.

And that was fortunate, for the next week was to bring the public announcement of my appointment, visits to Westminster, lunch with members of the Chapter, press interviews, and the beginning of a flood of letters which were to occupy every morning for the next month.

February

At this stage I still had doubts about being well enough to be installed as Dean in July, and I devised a thank-you letter which was a careful compromise – for those who could read between the lines – between gratitude and caution.

On 7th February I saw Doctor A for the last time. He discovered I was progressing as slowly as he had forecast, wished me luck and signed me off. I hoped he would add the frank and appealing words he used to a friend who has had a similar mystery illness: 'Of course you realise we haven't the faintest idea what's been wrong with you.' But he didn't.

A week later, working only in the morning, I was interviewed by *The Times*, and found myself back in the world where journalists wanted to know my views on the Bishop of Durham. Little had changed.

But things were looking more hopeful. Alison and I had not had a summer holiday the previous year and we planned to leave for Sicily on 18th February. With two days to go I went down with the fever I had earlier needed (for there is a type of viral infection which carries a high fever and tends to burn itself out more quickly), but this was a vicious form of 'flu. It seemed to focus in my lungs, gave me a fever for a week, and set me back at least two months. The rest of February was a write-off.

March

I was beginning to wake in the middle of the night feeling trapped: caught between a longing, prayerful, desperate demand to be well, and the discovery that each day brought the same discomfort, the same suffocating pressure in the lungs and sense of malaise. For months I had had a rash on my chest, mild in the morning, worse at night, which seemed to be an outward sign of something still wrong, but no one could tell me what. How could I let people go on assuming I would be well for Westminster? Even half a day in the office still knocked me out. Of course I was better, much better than six months ago, but not yet well.

It was then that my colleagues and churchwardens came to see me with an ultimatum. If I have not mentioned them before, and the miracle they worked in continuing to order the church's life with such smooth efficiency, that is because I am half-ashamed at having had it so lucky. No one could have had curates and churchwardens who showed more sympathetic understanding, kindness and tolerance. They told me bluntly that it was too late to get back into the life of Great St Mary's again with any sense of leadership; that I should do all I wished in Holy Week and Easter, go away to Sicily for a fortnight, come back for ten days and chair the Annual General Meeting, and then take virtually a month's sabbatical leave for which they would be financially responsible. The only concern in their minds was that I should be fully well for Westminster – and they weren't taking no for an answer. After a token show of resistance, I didn't argue.

It was a good Holy Week. By the grace of God I was able to play a full part each day, celebrating on Maundy Thursday, preaching on Good Friday, presiding on Easter Eve, and celebrating at the parish communion on Easter Day. Once before I thought I had turned the corner, but 'flu negated that. Now I knew I had done so and that eventually all would be well.

But I had still some things to learn.

April

Sadly, Sicily was a disaster. Visually it could not have looked more perfect: mimosa and fennel, wild lupins and fields of wild marigolds, even wild gladioli, and most of the English flowers of all our seasons blooming at once. But a combination of the hills, the sun, the journey and the sea mists knocked me for six, and I was reduced to sitting in the shade of the hotel garden painting endless bad water-colours of Taormina, nursing my aching lungs and limbs, and brooding on the unfairness of it all. Not all the time, but quite enough of it; dreading the decision to be made when we got home.

In fact no decision was necessary. The Sub-Dean of Westminster, with great understanding and patience, said they were prepared to fix a provisional date for my Installation and wait for it to be confirmed at the end of May.

As I write these words in the Dolomites, that is in ten days' time. And writing it down has helped me know my answer.

Forgive me if the detailing of such trivial events has made for wearisome reading; I can only say that the living of them proved even more wearisome, and that it has been an unforgettable year: unforgettable in the sense that I certainly would not choose to live through it again, but unforgettable too in the sense that I hope it will have proved to be a kind of watershed, for it has stopped me short in my tracks and offered me the chance of learning lessons which I need to know if I am to grow a little closer to what God wants me to be as I move into the last active job of my life.

Part II

May 1986

Looking back at what I have written, what emerges?

I may seem to have been critical, if only by implication, of the specialists. That is not my intention. They gave me their professional care, skill and attention. They were the first to admit that much research is still being done in the whole area of viral infections and at present there is often no real treatment other than rest.

Montaigne wrote, in one of his *Essays*:

> Medicine always claims that experience is the test of its operations. Plato therefore was right in saying that to become a true doctor, a man must have experienced all the illnesses he hopes to cure and all the accidents and circumstances he is to diagnose . . . Such a man I would trust. For the rest guide us like the person who paints seas, rocks and harbours while sitting at his table and sails his model of a ship in perfect safety. Throw him into the real thing, and he does not know where to begin.[17]

There is an important truth there, which all who care or counsel professionally need to hear; even so, there is a limit to the empathy one can expect from those whose experiences of illness is witnessing it in others.

But what of my need to be treated as a person, rather than a handful of symptoms? It is not individual doctors or specialists who are at fault so much as our whole modern approach to medicine, with its increasingly narrow specialisation. They can become victims of the system. A cynic might say that Doctor D, because he was retired, gave me a sense of worth because he had the time (and because I paid him) to do so; but in fact it was his grasp of the inter-relatedness of body and spirit which was so therapeutic, and while marvellous gains have been made by the use of modern technical apparatus, the growing concern with alternative medicine is not merely a 'fringe' interest but a deep instinctive awareness that what matters most, both in the doctor/patient relationship and in the process of healing, is in danger of being lost.

This emerges clearly in *The Healing Arts* (originally a documentary series on BBC television). By splitting human behaviour and human diseases into countless specialist fields, it increases the likelihood of no one being responsible for the whole person.

> By their very nature doctors deal with bits and pieces – microbes, hormone deficiencies or tumours – while patients experience illness as the disorder, disruption and possible disintegration of their ordinary lives. . . . Every healing art sees illness in its own terms. Patients need to remember that the illness is theirs and theirs alone.[18]

Reviewing this series in *The Times*, Andrew Rissik wrote:

> Doctors are not merely biological repair men, people

who know how we work and people who can twiddle knobs or replace faulty parts when they threaten to go wrong. A doctor must be a healer in the fullest, most spiritual sense, someone who accepts that human beings are congenitally lonely and dissatisfied but who may be able to reconcile them to the difficulties of their condition . . . to share the journey [of pain or anxiety or grief] with the patient.[19]

One of the more interesting experiments in healing is the new St Marylebone Centre for Healing and Counselling. This is an exciting attempt at a real partnership of religion and medicine, based on the conviction that the art of healing is enriched by learning from one another and practising alongside each other. A National Health Service surgery will work in the crypt centre alongside the church's own ministry of healing and counselling. The latter will consist of a team of people, priests and laity, counsellors and befrienders, who will be available to listen, to talk, to pray and lay on hands. There will also be space in the crypt for the practice of acupuncture and osteopathy, and there will be a music therapy unit. Here is an attempt to see the patient as a whole human being.

Another rare example of how doctors at the local level are resisting the pressure to treat a human being like a complex and temporarily (or permanently) disordered machine is in a group practice in Maidstone. A local GP has set up a Trust which seeks to understand illness in its whole human context; and to extend the art of healing through the use of therapists. Instead of depending wholly on the doctor to make them better, those suffering from chronic and debilitating diseases such as cancer, multiple sclerosis or coronary thrombosis, are invited to collaborate in their treatment, and take upon themselves some of the healing process, through counselling and various forms of therapy – art and music, modelling and eurythmy (movement therapy). It is a heartening attempt to recognise the uniqueness of each individual, and the positive healing potential we each have within us. It also encourages the seriously ill (through individual and group counselling) not to look on their illness purely in negative terms but to begin to come to terms with the fact of their own death.

*

Another matter on which I feel much more reluctant to write, is the effect my illness had on my family. So far as my son and daughter are concerned, what I would like to write would only embarrass them. Mark, at a local Sixth Form College in his first year of 'A' levels, was concerned and supportive in a completely unfussy way. For part of the year Sarah was away from home, and one of the hardest things for her was trying to share the joy of getting engaged in July with parents whose delight was muted, not by any lack of enthusiasm or pleasure, but by being for a while caught up in a world where the thought of a family wedding was hard to envisage.

The way husband and wife experience and respond to the vow to love and cherish each other 'in sickness and in health' is private to themselves, though observed by others. I am beginning now to understand the strain there was on Alison, and I shall always be grateful that a number of people understood this and quietly supported her.

Yet it is not enough to leave it there, in an understandable attempt to protect the private feelings of those you love. For that would be to side-step the important issue which confronts everyone facing serious illness: the fact that it is so destabilising that it can dissolve familiar roles and routines and disturb accepted relationships; and that this may stir up anxiety, anger and guilt on both sides.

Certainly, for Alison, there was anxiety and there was anger. In the early months, because no one really knew what was wrong, we were both anxious. It could have been a terminal illness or a very long-term one, and it was not really helped by those doctors (*not* our GP) who predicted that it would only be 'another few weeks'. Anger is not always very rational in choosing its targets, but it has to be targeted somewhere. Alison was angry with the consultants because they could not put a name to what was wrong with me, could not prescribe any drugs, and seemed not to be greatly interested or concerned. She was powerless to say anything as doctors rarely look beyond the patient or speak with those closest to them.

Gradually the possibility of a terminal illness receded, but for Alison there were still moments of panic which lasted for several months, especially in the small hours. For some while it was as if my brain had seized up and I would find myself groping for familiar words, and failing to listen or take in what I was told. I was both aware and unaware of this: too withdrawn into myself and too emotionally diminished to do much about it. Alison had to choose whether to share the anxiety and the pain with the few friends who were ready to listen or to batten down the hatches and carry on. Partly because she is a naturally private person, and partly because she was afraid that if she once let go she might not be able to carry on, she did the latter.

For the same reason, Alison found it hard to know how much to share with me. Suddenly everything devolved on her, all the jobs we had previously done together:

41

gardening, mowing the lawn, dealing with people, dealing with the family. It was no longer possible to discuss anything in the way we had been used to, and it is hard to know how much to share when you are getting little response. Nor was it easy to share her anxieties with friends who called, not even the clergy, for they tended only to focus on her through me.

Alison, like me, learned more about the difficult art of visiting the sick: the importance of giving of yourself, of being interested, *really* interested, when you ask how someone is; not coming when you are tired; not staying too long; not sharing your own experience of illness; sharing an item of common interest. She respected the need people had to ask her how I was: they had a right to know. What angered her was that, although we hid nothing and were always open with such information as we had, the rumours flew around. Perhaps the medical profession is partly to blame. Doctors tend to withhold information which it should be routine to share, sometimes because they have no time to cope with the difficulties that may follow if they do so, but often because they are not always good at communicating with people who have little understanding of how their bodies function. And this can create a kind of medical filter on facts about our own minds and bodies.

One of the minor problems about looking after someone you love at home is to know whether to go out, sit with them, or simply try to carry on life as before: it is a constant juggling act. The worst points, surprisingly, came when we went away – Stratford, Devon, Sicily – for the instant cure you feel it may produce doesn't happen; and then, perversely, though you have longed for a change of routine, you long even more to be back among familiar things and familiar faces.

Looking back now, Alison cannot remember what she read, what kind of winter it was, what happened at Christmas. There is a kind of amnesia, a blotting out of those difficult months which for me remain so vivid. But for her, too, there were compensations, small but important redemptive features: the growth into a more adult relationship with our children, with whom she shared a lot; the enormous support we both received from friends at Great St Mary's; a new appreciation of the good things in our lives as she looked back and, hopefully, forward. And a very tentative but new understanding of what the relatives of those in the local hospice (where she worked as a volunteer) go through, and a new respect for the way different individuals cope, sometimes in very personal and unconventional ways.

The effect of my illness on the wider family of the church is not easy to assess. Untypically and luckily, I had colleagues. Services went on; pastoral needs were met. Providentially, the church council had planned a year on the meaning of ministry, that is to say, the ministry of the baptised in a city-centre church. The talking now became irrelevant: the question was what you actually did when the vicar was totally out of action. A number of lay-people discovered in themselves a potential to act, not just in making decisions previously wrongly felt to be the exclusive prerogative of the clergy, but also as pastors.

*

For myself, I had to question my perception of God as he can be known in the bad times as well as the good, and in particular go on to relate my experience to my understanding of the Cross. Certain theological books have an effect out of all proportion to their size. One which may become a classic is W. H. Vanstone's *The*

Stature of Waiting.[20] In it he describes the gospel accounts of Jesus' life and ministry as falling into two distinct phases: one of dynamic, inexhaustible activity interspersed with times of silence and prayer; and a second, contrasting phase of passivity. The turning point comes in Gethsemane where Judas hands Jesus over to forces beyond his control and the Passion has begun. No longer is Jesus the active initiator, free to go where he will: now his hands are tied and he is at the disposal of others, the one who patiently endures, not the one who *does*, but the one who is *done to*. Now he is at the mercy of those who try him, flog and scourge and crucify him. He cannot even carry his own cross, but is waited on, served, by one who happens to be passing by.

Vanstone then takes this pattern of the active and passive sides of the life of Jesus and relates it to the pattern of our own lives. As we grow older we increasingly become those for whom things are done or to whom things are done, often because of the handicaps of illness or advancing old age. In many eloquent passages Vanstone argues the value and the importance of being and receiving, of learning to endure patiently yet creatively, of what he calls 'the stature of waiting'. And in a chapter called 'The God who Waits' he shows that God himself has chosen to become a passive receiver and to place himself in our hands. He argues that this is so from what we observe in Jesus, whose way of living and dying reveals the nature of the Father. God is seen to be like one who heals and sets free and washes his followers' feet, and also like one who suffers and endures the worst we can do to him. For in fact Jesus *chooses* his Passion, he goes voluntarily to Jerusalem, he lets himself be robbed of all his outward freedom. For he knows that this is the only way for Love to act. He has to show that God's way

44

is not to coerce men and women by force or limit their freedom, but to allow them to do with him what they will, and – as patiently as the father in the story of the Prodigal Son – to wait and to endure with an unchanging love.

Nowhere is Jesus more powerful than in his passive suffering on the Cross. Nowhere does he show more clearly the truth of the passive, suffering God whose hands are tied by love.

Vanstone therefore believes that the image of God is to be seen in us – as it was in Jesus – equally in our *active* lives, in our work and our creativity, and in our *passive* lives, by the way in which we accept and respond to the things that are done to us. Or indeed, as we grow old, or as we endure illness, by our response to the things which are done for us. This means that those forced to be inactive by lack of work or handicap or illness or old age need not feel they are of any less value as human beings. Rather, this time can be seen as a true and creative sharing in the nature of a God who himself became powerless and vulnerable.

Richard Holloway, meditating on Vanstone's book asks:

> What if the thing we are meant to learn about God is that he is a waiting, suffering God who is acted upon rather than acts? Is there some truth here that we've lost? Are we so upset about suffering because we are so busy and activist and obsessed with solving problems that we have not waited long enough to expose ourselves to the scandalous truth about the meaning of suffering? Is suffering, submission to necessity, the carrier of redemption? And is redemption experienced

within the suffering rather than in being rescued *from* the suffering?[21]

On the Good Friday before I was ill I preached about the meaning of the stature of waiting: now I had the chance to experience its truth. Waiting on God (which Simone Weil said was the most important thing of all) is hard when you are dispirited by illness. But part of waiting on God, learning to be passive in a way creative for your inner life, is not a question of *thinking* about God, but of growing in stillness. It has to do with prayer, and with that interior silence which may come from listening to music or from the simple contemplation of the world about you.

I have written of the solitude of illness; of the difficulty of avoiding that natural self-obsession of the invalid, the nagging anxiety, the self-pity brought on by your daily discomfort. And yet there are compensations. If you are a priest, for a while it is not possible to spin round the parish like a whirling dervish. You are no longer conditioned by time and people and events. You can let go, and begin to observe the world around you with its own different kind of rhythm of birth and death and rebirth, and learn again the truth you have once known – perhaps on retreat or on holiday – but forgotten: that in the words of Jeremy Taylor, 'There should be in the soul halls of space, avenues of leisure, and high porticos of silence, where God walks.'[22]

For there is a different kind of passivity, one that is not necessarily forced upon us by illness or old age, but one that is chosen because it goes to the very heart of what it means to be a follower of Christ – and certainly the very heart of what it means to be a priest. Stillness is a rare and precious quality. 'Nothing in all creation', wrote the fourteenth-century German mystic, Meister Eckhart (and the words now hang in my study), 'is so like God as stillness.' Stillness has to do with seeing, with the opening of our eyes to another dimension, to the mystery of God that lies all about us; and it is the specific task of the priest 'to keep the mystery of God present to man'.

Bishop John Taylor, in *The Go-Between God*, says this about the Holy Spirit as the giver of vision:

> The Holy Spirit is the invisible third party who stands between me and the other, making us mutually aware. Supremely and primarily he opens my eyes to Christ. But he also opens my eyes to the brother in Christ, or the fellow man, or the point of need, or the heart-breaking brutality and the equally heart-breaking beauty of the world. He is the giver of that vision without which the people perish. We commonly speak about the Holy Spirit as the source of power. But in fact he enables us not by making us supernaturally strong but by opening our eyes.[23]

Part of that vision relates to the world of nature, our deepened awareness 'of the heart-breaking brutality and the equally heart-breaking beauty of the world'. I will come to the brutality by and by: for the moment consider its beauty:

> What marks off . . . the deep ones from the superficial . . . [is] their sense of wonder, awe, and joy before what is there for all to behold; the fact that we are alive, that there is anything at all . . . This sense of awe and wonder occurs when one is *struck* by the fact that I am, and that I am I, that a tree is itself, that there is anything at all.[24]

So writes Paul van Buren. Not only is each one of us, in

the Psalmist's words, 'fearfully and wonderfully made', a mysterious complex of matter and spirit created with a detailed precision we should find breathtaking, but there is about us, if only we have eyes to see, a creation of such spectacular profusion, spendthrift richness and absurd detail, as to make us catch our breath in astonished wonder. 'October 20th: St Luke's summer. Trees have the power to startle me more and more.' So wrote Philip Toynbee in that remarkable diary he kept the year before he died.[25] And a hundred and fifty years earlier Blake had written: 'The tree which moves some to tears of joy is in the eyes of others only a green thing that stands in the way.' He also wrote to his friend George Richmond: 'I sometimes look at the knot in a piece of wood until I am frightened at it.'

Frightened: awestruck: full of Job-like wonder at the scale on which the Creator works. 'The place from which all spirituality must begin' wrote Bishop Ian Ramsey, 'is the created world around us'.[26]

My understanding of the priesthood begins there: with the vision of a world which is God's world because behind it, within it, informing it (if we have eyes to see), is the fact of God's saving love, so that the world is not merely beautiful, it is sacramental, incarnational. Everything in creation can become the sign and means of God's presence if we have eyes to see.

Monica Furlong, in her book *Travelling In*, writes, 'Priests are justified only by their powers of being and seeing.'[27] 'Being' and 'seeing': I must be able to carve out of my life a space for prayer and silence and simple contemplation which alone enables me to give attention to people and things, really observe them, really listen, instead of conveying the message that I too am hard-pressed, busy and anxious.

I have always loved a passage from Kierkegaard's *Christian Discourses*:

> But what does this mean, what have I to do, or what sort of effort is it that can be said to seek or pursue the Kingdom of God? Shall I try to get a job suitable to my talents and powers in order thereby to exert an influence? No, thou shalt first seek God's kingdom. Shall I then give all my fortune to the poor? No, thou shalt first seek God's kingdom. Shall I then go out to proclaim his teaching to the world? No, thou shalt first seek God's kingdom. But then in a sense it is nothing I shall do. Yes, certainly, in a certain sense it is nothing; thou shalt in the deepest sense make thyself nothing, become nothing before God, learn to keep silent; in this silence is the beginning, which is, first to seek God's kingdom.[28]

And there is a second passage in which Kierkegaard asks how Christ managed to live 'without anxiety for the next day', when he must have known from the beginning of his public ministry how his life would end. It was, he says, because 'he had Eternity with him in the day that is called today, hence the next day had no power over him, it had no existence for him'.[29]

That is all of a piece with the teaching of the eighteenth-century French priest, Jean-Pierre de Caussade and what he called 'the sacrament of the present moment'; or of Meister Eckhart, who once said that holiness 'consists in doing the next thing you have to do, doing it with your whole heart, and finding delight in doing it'. Or with some words of the playwright, Dennis Potter, in an unpublished Lent talk for the BBC:

> We were able, once upon a time, to live out our days

minute by minute. One of the strangest, most heart-ening, and indeed most irritatingly exhausting things about children, and therefore of what we ourselves once were, is their ability to live almost entirely in the present tense.

To do that, of course, presupposes an immense trust in the order of things. Apply it not to a child, but to an adult aware of the world and of his or her responsi-bilities, and the first thing you notice about such a mode of response is the immense degree of concentration and sustained *attention* that it implies.

Yet it is perhaps not quite so difficult. Whenever we play games, or act, or sing, or dance, or make love, we are outside 'normal' time, we are in the cauldron of the actual minute, and we have suspended or evaded the claims of any other moment except *this* one. When we are frightened, when we are in pain, when we are excited, and when we are greatly moved, the world stands still. Once again – to our delight or not – all things are as new.[30]

'He had eternity with him the day that is called today.' I have loved to quote it: and I have rarely achieved it. Forced now to be inactive, perhaps this truth will once again take root in me. Perhaps here is one of the answers I have been groping after as I ask God why he has stopped me dead in my tracks and interrupted a busy ministry in full flow; and why my healing is so slow.

*

I hope, too, that I have come to understand a little more of the inner world and its complexities: that world of inner consciousness, which is daily influenced and shaped by our relationships, our work, what we read and watch and hear, and what follows from all these things: our doubts and fears, our hopes and expectations, our sadnesses and joys. As Father Gerard Hughes writes in his fine book, *God of Surprises*:

This inner world is unique in each of us, mysterious and incommunicable even to ourselves in its complexity . . . Although we cannot understand this hidden world, we know that it holds the key to our happiness and our personality . . . [and] if we allow ourselves time to think, we become increasingly conscious of the complexity of our inner life, of the mystery of it, and of the layers upon layers of consciousness within us.

Yet only if we can take time, without guilt or fear, to explore this inner world of the self shall we encounter God, 'the God of mystery, the God of surprises, whose Spirit is at work in our spirit in a manner unique to each individual'.[31]

There is a poem by Caryll Houselander about a young man

who lives in a world of progress.
He used to worship a God
who was kind to him.
This God had a long white beard,
He lived in the clouds,
but all the same
He was close to the solemn child
who had secretly
shut him up, in a picture book.

The poet tells how the young man works twelve hours a day and lives 'in a lodging house, that is not a home'. After a dreary life, he grows old and soon will die; and the poem ends:

If he had only known
that the God in the picture book,
is not an old man in the clouds
but the seed of life in his soul,
the man would have lived.
And his life would have flowered
with the flower of limitless joy.

But he does not know,
and in him
the Holy Ghost
is a poor little bird
in a cage,
who never sings,
and never opens his wings,
yet never, never
desires to be gone away.[32]

*

If I am to face the deeper questions about my ministry
and my illness, and how something apparently so negative
and destructive may have been used creatively (or, better,
redemptively) by God to stop me in my tracks, then I
must tease out the implications of Vanstone's *The Stature
of Waiting*, Hughes's *God of Surprises* and Caryll Houselander's God who 'never, never desires to be gone away'.

For God may be wholly Other, the Creator who is
mysterious and unimaginable, of whom St Paul can write:
'How unsearchable his judgements, how untraceable his
ways! Who knows the mind of the Lord? Who has been
his counsellor?'[33] But he is also the God revealed in Jesus
Christ, whose Spirit is even now within me and who
desires only that I shall grow in the knowledge of his love.
And if God can be known so intimately, then I must rid
my mind of the unhelpful image of a distant Creator to

52

whom I must beg for my prayer to be heard.

Much of the Old Testament, with its tales of human violence and divine wrath, many of which are inevitably read in our churches out of context, simply confirms our immature concept of God as a creator who is all-powerful and a predestinator who is all-knowing, who will act with kindness towards those who do his will, and punish those who resist him. Yet what the New Testament proclaims, in all that we mean when we say 'Jesus Christ', is an event so singular and so revealing that it can only be compared to a new act of creation. In Jesus Christ, 'the new man', 'the second Adam', we see both God's human face, and man as he is meant to be.

'No one has ever seen God;' writes St John, 'it is the only Son, he who is nearest to the Father's heart, who has made him known.'[34] And he has made him known in the only terms we can understand: in human terms, as the man Jesus Christ. His every word and action is radiated by his knowledge of the Father, and so we can now say that God is like a man who heals the sick and loves the sinner; who takes a basin and towel and washes his disciples' feet; who, when nailed to a cross, forgives those who are nailing him there. Jesus knows the Father to be wholly Love, and that to be reconciled to God is to be caught up into 'a love that will not let us go'. He knows that we are made in God's likeness, made to reflect that likeness in living a life for others, for only in true self-giving love (part of which is the worship and praise of God) shall we find our fulfilment.

I have longed to be used to free people from their innate fear and guilt, from an image of God which, for example, causes so many patients in hospices or cancer wards to ask 'Why has God done this to me?' That is not the God of Jesus Christ. Certainly God is rock-like in his concern for justice, righteousness and the truth of his Kingdom, but he draws us into that Kingdom by his compassion, not by force. Loving us into being, he will (if we trust him) love us into eternal life as we respond, however feebly and haltingly, to the Life within us, that Life – to use the vivid metaphor in St John's Gospel – which 'wells up like a spring inside us'. Dennis Potter writes:

I came to understand that God . . . is not an unctuous palliative, or a super-pill, or a sugary abstraction, but . . . someone present in the quick of being, one's own being, and in the present tense itself, in existence as it exists, in the fibre and the pulse of the world, and in the minute-by-minute drama of an ever-continuing, ever-poised, ever-accessible creation.[35]

To believe that 'God was in Christ' is to believe something very startling indeed. It is to claim with Bishop Michael Ramsey that 'God is Christ-like and in him is no unChristlikeness at all'.[36] It is to stand with Dame Cicely Saunders, founder of St Christopher's Hospice, when – out of her years of experience at the bedside of dying patients – she can say:

Surely all the hard things that have happened to anyone in his creation have happened to God himself. As any mother, seeing a child suffer is suffering herself, so the Father of everyone has received all the sorrow and pain himself . . . and the presence of Jesus in history was the presence of God as he has always been and will always be.[37]

What the New Testament claims is that Jesus cannot be properly understood unless in saying his name you say 'God'; and that neither can God be known, not properly known, unless in saying his name you say 'Jesus'. And that neither can be known unless you use the word 'Love'. In Jesus Christ, in a way we cannot comprehend but which our heart tells us is true, there is a uniting of divine action and human response. In him we see what God is like; in him we see what each person is meant to be. But Jesus Christ does not only change our idea of what God is and what we might become: he also changes our idea of what love is. For 'the love of God in Jesus Christ our Lord' is not a love which is soft and yielding and emotional. This love is diamond-hard and costly: it is a giving of yourself to others; it is a refusal to hate, whatever the cost; it is a refusal to be moved from what you know in your heart to be good and true and right. Love is quite often a kind of dying. It demands obedience and loyalty, and it may well encompass anguish, pain and even death.

And so the heart of this disclosure of God as Love is in the event to which the whole of the earthly life of Jesus inexorably moves: the Cross. It is the implicit claim of the New Testament writers (to quote John Austin Baker's familiar words) that 'the crucified Jesus is the only accurate picture of God the world has ever seen'.[38] Or, in Bonhoeffer's words: 'To be a Christian . . . means participation in the suffering of God in the life of the world.' 'Only a suffering God can help.'[39] It is no good having some ready-made idea of God and then trying to make Jesus Christ fit into it. For if we take seriously the idea of God reconciling the world to himself by revealing himself in Jesus Christ, then we must be willing to have our understanding of God totally and irrevocably changed by what is revealed.

It is indeed a strange and unlikely truth that we Christians have to give to the world. Most people would like to think there is a God, a creative power behind and within the universe, and that this power is personal and loving. But they find it hard to relate that truth to the pain and unfairness of life. The world doesn't feel or look as if it is made by a God who is love. Yet it is exactly at that point – where what we long for and what we experience do not seem to fit or make sense – that God answers us with his Word. His Word made flesh. 'Jesus . . . contracts the immensities and focusses the infinite. He is God focussed to a point.'[40] God is not indifferent. God immerses himself in his creation and is born a man, one exactly like ourselves, and at the crib in Bethlehem the image of God as a power to be afraid of, as somehow speaking through the blind forces of nature, that image dies. We see God in human terms: not up there, somewhere far off and over against us, but here, made flesh, for us and with us and in our midst.

Only the Passion and death of Jesus can reconcile those two apparently irreconcilable truths: that God is in love with us, and that at some point in our lives we all experience suffering, pain and dereliction. Either God was not in Christ and the Cross is the ultimate symbol of all the meaninglessness that can destroy us, the absence of God, the triumph of the secular powers. Or God was in Christ and the Cross is the final word of a God who shares the pain and the dirt, the loneliness and the weakness, even the frightening sense of desolation and the death we may be called upon to experience ourselves. That was the audacious claim of the first Christians, that God is now revealed as the one who pours himself out in love, a serving, foot-washing, crucified God, whose love cannot be altered or diminished.

But we need to walk a little warily here. To say that 'God is like Jesus' is not to say that 'Jesus is like God'. The latter would mean that the One whose glory no man can look upon and live, the God of Gods and the Lord of Lords, is reduced to human dimensions, and that cannot be so. But to say that God is like Jesus is to believe that the One whom we call God chose to reveal as much as we need to know of his nature in the only terms we can understand, and that 'the crucified Jesus is the only accurate picture of God the world has ever seen'. 'Some of us believe', wrote Julian of Norwich, 'that God is all-powerful and *may* do everything; and that he is all-wise and *can* do everything; but as for believing that he is all-Love and will do everything, there we hold back. In my view nothing hinders God's lovers more than the failure to understand this.'[41]

If the Cross is a declaration of God's love as in Christ he identifies himself with us at every point, it is also a declaration of God's forgiveness. If I were to sum up in a sentence why I am a Christian (let alone a priest) I would say that it is because I believe in the Passion of Jesus Christ and the compassion of God. Passion from the Latin *passio*, meaning 'to suffer'; compassion from *cum passio* meaning 'to suffer alongside'. I see and experience a world which has pain and suffering at its centre; I believe in a God who loves each of us beyond our imagining; and in a gospel which brings the two together at a place called Calvary.

Yet there is a feeble gospel and there is a powerful gospel. The feeble gospel looks back to Jesus as our model, our example, and is much concerned with moral injunctions. It sees his teaching as a fine set of ideals at which to aim. It may not do much harm but it has no power to change your life: it is a faith built in sand which leaves you untouched at the centre and vulnerable and exposed when life knocks you flat on your face. The powerful gospel, on the other hand, has at its centre the Cross and the Passion of Jesus and the compassion of

57

God. It speaks of these truths both as historical and as present realities. It speaks of forgiveness and of dying, of resurrection and new life.

For me, and I guess for many, that gospel is something I both fear and long for. My life has contained no sudden blinding conversion, rather a series of small but undeniable glimpses of the reality of God's love, and the powerful, constantly repeated, small but utterly real experiences of forgiveness and new life. To follow Christ is to know in your bones the truth of this new life made possible by the Cross and Resurrection, and be seized by a vision of a world turned topsy-turvy; a world in which greatness lies in the service of others and love means the giving of yourself; in which the good will often be crucified and glory lies in being prepared to suffer; in which if you wish to find your life you must learn to lose it. It is a world (a Kingdom) whose currency is compassion, forgiveness, reconciliation and trust; and that other worldly world in which we live out our lives will think it foolishness. Nevertheless at every Eucharist we unite ourselves with the one who identified himself with the bread which was taken, given thanks for, broken and shared.

> You are the body of Christ [writes St Augustine]: that is to say, in you and through you the work of the Incarnation must go forward. You are meant to incarnate in your lives the theme of your adoration – you are to be taken, consecrated, broken and distributed, that you may be the means of grace and vehicles of the Eternal Charity.[42]

I have understood my priesthood as an invitation to others to share that vision, trying in the pulpit or in encounters with individuals to find the words which will make sense of it, acting it out day by day, and week by week, in the drama of the Eucharist. And central to the truth that others in their turn have shown me is that 'eucharist' means 'thanksgiving', that in giving thanks for the bread and wine we are asserting that thanksgiving is the central and most important element in the Christian response to life. 'Thank God at all times for everything,'[43] writes St Paul; and again, 'give thanks, whatever happens'.[44] 'It is our duty and our joy, at all times and in all places, to give you thanks and praise . . .'

When Father Christopher Bryant, Superior of the Society of St John the Evangelist, died, his obituarist wrote of him:

> Perhaps the image for us all to bear in mind while coming to terms with losing him is one familiar to many who turned to him in trouble. He would listen and share the pain; then, leaning slightly forward with a gentle smile, he would enquire: 'Have you tried *thanking* God for it?'[45]

And William Law, in his *Serious Call to a Holy and Devout Life*, said this:

> If anyone would tell you the shortest, surest way to all happiness, all perfection, he would tell you to make a rule to yourself to thank and praise God for *everything* that happens to you. For it is certain that whatever seeming calamity happens to you, if you thank and praise God for it, you turn it into a blessing. Could you therefore work miracles, you could not do more for yourself than by the thankful spirit, for it heals with a word spoken, and turns all that it touches into happiness.[46]

To live like this, whatever life brings, in good days and bad, to live positively and creatively, trying to thank God for it all, is to enter more deeply into the meaning of the

Cross. I have preached as much, often, choosing my words with care.

But when it came to the crunch, when I was physically weak and in pain, then at times I simply could not do it. It was not that the beliefs which shaped my life had proved unreliable or untrue, but rather that I was, perhaps for the first time, experiencing the darkness, which though it takes many forms, comes to all of us. I was for a while not only utterly dependent on others but shut up, imprisoned, in myself.

*

How then did I try to keep faith with this God, who is truly the ground of my being, when he seemed so deaf to my desire to be healed?

In three ways. First, by this very dependence on others. I let others do the praying for me. It was not that I lost my faith, but rather that I fell back with relief on the truth of St Paul's words about the body of Christ, and its different members each with their different gifts and functions. In a perfectly real and valid sense other members were doing for me what I found hard to do, praying and caring and breaking bread together; and I had to learn what it means to receive and to be served in *this* aspect of one's life as well as in others. This truth of mutual interdependence is yet another facet of the 'stature of waiting', of the enforced passivity of the sick and the old, the muddled and the mentally ill, who temporarily or permanently cannot act for themselves but can know that others are praying on their behalf. And that, too, is a kind of keeping faith.

Secondly, when I could I tried very simply to pray the Psalms, with their extraordinary insight into the human heart, together with their constant refrain of confidence and trust. The Psalmist looks forward to the God revealed by Jesus and shows how ancient and how contemporary are both the dread and the hope which inform us.

And thirdly, I tried to repeat the simplest of phrases, from the Psalms and elsewhere, which affirm the truth that never for one single moment can we be cut off from the God 'in whom we live and move and have our being'. This, as I have said, is not to diminish God who is mystery, unimaginable in his power and majesty. For part of the mystery is that he is also in the heart of every one of us, drawing us to himself with a love we cannot yet begin to grasp. Such words as God's words to Israel: 'You are mine . . . you are precious in my eyes and . . . I love you,'[47] or the Psalmist's 'In the hour of fear: I will put my trust in you',[48] or those words from Hebrews: 'God himself has said, "I will never leave you or desert you"; and so I can take courage and say, "The Lord is my helper, I will not fear; what can man do to me?" '[49] were phrases I tried to dwell on, hoping their truth would become a deep part of me.

I hinted earlier that, even in the dark times, I never experienced that God had abandoned me, nor was I seriously depressed. But I can certainly understand how this can happen and a little of what it must feel like. In a depressive illness there is a sense of loss and diminishment, the feeling of being trapped in a blackness which distorts both past and future; of being isolated, cut off from your family and friends, any faith in God lost in a sense of despair, so that with Job you cry out:

And now the life in me trickles away
   days of grief have gripped me.
At night-time, sickness saps my bones,
   I am gnawed by wounds that never sleep.[50]

61

Depressive illnesses are not my subject: they take many forms, and doctors still disagree as to their origin and their treatment. And yet almost always there is in true depression a basis of anger, and it may be that the only 'religious' feeling possible is the attempt to tap and understand some of that repressed resentment and anger and direct it at God. Once again that will only be possible if our understanding of God has progressed from one of fear to one of childlike trust, confidence and love. 'Unless you become like little children . . .' The God of Jesus Christ offers himself as the butt of people's anger. He knows what it is to be strung up on a cross, spat and railed at and abused. If we are going to come to terms with our inner selves at any but the most superficial level, then being honest with God (which includes being angry with God) may be the starting point. God is not shocked by our rage or resentment. And he alone can absorb it and from it bring something creative.

So, once again, that which has most to say to the sick or suffering person – in this case the depressive – is the Cross of Christ. That Cross shows us at our most hateful and destructive: equally it shows God in Christ at his most forgiving and creative. Whatever we do or fail to do, whatever we feel or fail to feel, though the heavens seem barred against us when we try to pray and no answer comes, yet there is no diminution of his love. 'If I go down to hell thou art there also.'[51]

It is hard for a person with severe depression, someone who may be suicidal, to have any sense that God is with them in the darkness. Here, too, you cannot act by yourself. Just as in my own worst time of sickness – even though it was more of a long-drawn-out despondency – I needed to depend on the prayers and sympathetic understanding of others, so someone suffering from a depressive illness depends on that quality of compassionate understanding which does not dismiss their black despair as nonsense, or treat it as something of which one should be ashamed.

Often people who are ill have told me that they seem to have lost their faith, when what they mean is that they no longer find it possible to pray. At least I was able to go on praying a little, in however diminished a way. Many can't. I do not simply mean a felt awareness of God, for at the best of times and for the best of people there may be long periods when prayer means persisting with little or no feeling, no awareness of God's presence, when it is more a wanting God than a perceiving him. I mean when it seems impossible to pray at all – to give thanks, to ask for forgiveness, to wait on God in silence, to hold up others in his presence. But this is more often a loss of physical (and therefore spiritual) well-being rather than a loss of faith.

One of those who have written most perceptively about prayer, and not least about prayer in periods of darkness and apparent unbelief, is Neville Ward. Somewhere he writes that there will be times when we are reduced to seeing light nowhere but in the face of Christ, that the one solitary fact I can attempt to be thankful for in my present state is that the world of which I am part 'contains Christ's history and presence. But that's the whole point.' That is not to cease to pray: it is to maintain my relationship with the God revealed in Christ in other ways, even if only by repeating affirmations of the nearness and the love of God which I cannot feel. In a recent poem R. S. Thomas speaks of

> Prayers like gravel
> flung at the sky's

63

> window, hoping to attract
> > the loved one's
> attention . . .

I would
> have refrained long since
> > but that peering once
> through my locked fingers
> I thought that I detected
> > the movement of a curtain.[52]

*

But I need to come back to the centrality of the Cross as
the sign of God's unquenchable love, his involvement in
our suffering. For my illness, tiresome as it was, was as
nothing compared with that of many who are desperately
afflicted and whose faith in a loving God is tested to
the limit: people like my former broadcasting colleague,
Robert Foxcroft, who after a courageous battle against
cancer, shared with millions through his 1985 Lent talks
on radio, died a few months later on New Year's Day.

There is a novel by Peter de Vries called *The Blood of
the Lamb*, about the grief of a father at the death of his
child from leukaemia. It is a strange, persuasive mixture
of humour, pain and rage. When he first learns of his
daughter's illness he spends more and more time in the
local church, engaged in a dialogue with the God in whom
he cannot quite bring himself to believe.

'Are God and Herod then one?'
'What do you mean?'
'The slaughter of the Innocents. Who creates a
perfect blossom to crush it? Children dying in one
building, the mice used in research in the next. It's all
the same to Him who marks the fall of the sparrow.'

'I forgive you.'
'I cannot say the same.'

Later, on another visit to the church, he goes to the little side chapel of St Jude, Patron of Lost Causes and Hopeless Cases.

I lit a candle. I was alone in the church. The gentle flames wavered and shattered in a mist of tears spilling from my eyes as I sank to the floor.

'I do not ask that she be spared to me, but that her life be spared to her. Or give us a year. We will spend it as we have the last, missing nothing. We will mark the dance of every hour between the snowdrop and the snow: crocus to tulip to violet to iris to rose. . . . When winter comes, we will let no snow fall ignored. . . . We will feed the plain birds that stay to cheer us through the winter, and when spring returns we shall be the first out, to catch the snowdrops' first white whisper in the wood. All this we ask, with the remission of our sins, in Christ's name. Amen.'

So begins a time of living to the hilt, squeezing from every moment of each day all it has to give. Sometimes, when alone, he gives way to rage and despair.

Dead-drunk, yet cold-sober, he wandered out to the garden in the cool of the evening awaiting the coming of the Lord. No such advent taking place, he shook his fist at the sky and cried, 'If you won't save her from pain, at least let me keep her from fear!' A brown thrush began his evening note, the ever-favoured, unendurable woodsong. I snatched up a rock from the ground and stoned it from the tree.

Later, he falls to wondering why other parents in the

children's ward chatter of this and that and never speak of the grief that burns within them. 'Rage and despair are indeed carried about in the heart, but privately, to be let out on special occasions, like savage dogs for exercise, occasions in solitude when God is cursed, birds stoned from the trees or the pillow hammered in darkness.' (I am reminded of some words of Flaubert: 'Human language is like a cracked kettle on which we beat out tunes for bears to dance to, when all the time we are longing to move the stars to pity.')

On his daughter's birthday, the father takes a beauti-fully iced birthday cake to the hospital. He learns on his arrival that she has come down with a severe throat infection and, having no resistance, has died.

> The nurse stepped outside a moment, and I moved quickly from the foot of the bed round to the side, whispering in our moment alone: 'The Lord bless thee and keep thee. The Lord make his face shine upon thee, and be gracious unto thee. The Lord lift up his countenance upon thee, and give thee peace.' I touched her stigmata one by one, the prints of the needles on her hands (where the blood had been given), the wound in the breast (where the sample of marrow had been taken). I caressed the now bald, perfectly shaped head. I bent to kiss the cheeks and the breasts that would now never be fulfilled: 'Oh, my lamb!'

There follows a great bursting anger against God. He returns to the church still clutching the birthday cake, and throws it with all his strength at the figure of Christ on the Cross outside the central doorway.

> It was miracle enough that the pastry should reach its target at all . . . the more so that it should land squarely,

just beneath the crown of thorns. Then through scalded eyes I seemed to see the hands free themselves of the nails and move slowly towards the soiled face. Very slowly, but very deliberately, with infinite patience, the icing was wiped from the eyes and flung away.

At Calvary God in Christ invites us to vent our anger and our rage upon him in order that we may discover in him a love that is stronger than our hate. And in the final few pages of the novel there is a kind of hope, a glimmering of redemption. The anger is still there, the question 'Why?' has not been answered, and yet he has learned through his daughter and those associated with her during her final months the meaning of compassion: the sharing of suffering. He reverses the words of Jesus, 'Blessed are they that mourn for they shall be comforted' into 'Blessed are they that comfort, for they have mourned.' And in the last words of the book the father meets his daughter's teacher, Miss Halsey:

> 'Some poems are long, some are short. She was a short one,' Miss Halsey said. Again the throb of compassion rather than the breath of consolation: the recognition of how long, how long is the mourner's bench upon which we sit, arms linked in undeluded friendship, all of us, brief links, ourselves, in the eternal pity.[53]

I cannot believe in a God who arbitrarily selects who shall live and who shall die – or who for some unimaginable reason expresses his love for us by removing from this world children by means of cancer.

The word 'mystery', when applied to God and the things of God, does not mean a puzzle we may one day be clever enough to solve but a truth beyond the limit of our present finite minds, and part of the mystery we have to live with is that the laws of nature operate without respect for persons, and often in what seems to us a cruel fashion. But a world with no such freedom and no such dependable and consistent laws of cause and effect would be far more horrific and dangerous. And part of the mystery of the Christian God is that he is not (as we imagine) the one who *orders* the fall of the sparrow, or the cancerous growth, any more than he *orders* the torture of a victim in some unknown prison cell, but the one who is truly incarnate in his creation. He was incarnate once and uniquely in Jesus Christ, but he is incarnate also, if we have eyes to see, in his suffering, struggling creatures.

This is the most important and miraculous opening of our eyes by the Holy Spirit: when our eyes are opened to the living Christ who encounters us in and through one another. In part of a poem called 'Christus', Monica Furlong writes:

> In night
> day
> pain
> joy
> I find you, and I see
> You in my lover,
> Child,
> Friend,
> All who love
> Me.
>
> In beggars,
> tramps,
> thieves,
> tarts,
> I'm supposed to find
> Your face

I have not quite
Yet
Managed
Such grace.

But in sick,
sad,
old,
bereaved,
I do sometimes guess
At your
glory,
majesty,
beauty,
tenderness.[54]

I shall always remember visiting Mother Teresa's Home for the Dying in Calcutta and being shown round by the sister-in-charge, Sister Luke. The dying lie on thin palliasses of straw, the men in one section of the extended ward, the women and children in the other. Between the two wards is a small cubicle with a plastic curtain drawn across the front of it. Just before I reached the home an old woman had been brought in from the streets in a filthy condition. She was barely recognisable as human.

'Come and see,' said Sister Luke, and took me across to the curtained-off trough. She drew back the curtain. The trough was filled with a few inches of water, in which was lying the stick-like body of the old woman. Two Missionaries of Charity were gently washing her clean and comforting her at the same time. Above the trough, stuck to the wall, was a simple notice containing four words: 'The body of Christ'. It is an image I can never forget.

Nor is it right to raise false hopes that prayer will of itself achieve what medical science cannot achieve. Prayer is about attuning yourself to the love of God, who wills all that is good for us, but it does not override the progress of the cancer cell. Thirty years ago, in his Gifford lectures, Professor John Macmurray drew this contrast:

The maxim of illusory religion runs: 'Fear not; trust in God and he will see that none of the things you fear will happen to you'; that of real religion, on the contrary, is: 'Fear not, the things that you are afraid of are quite likely to happen to you, but they are nothing to be afraid of'.[55]

Prayer, then is about daring to make the inward journey, and takes the form of penitence, praise and thanksgiving. And yet it is about asking too: asking for my healing, or for Bill or Mary's healing, because it is natural to ask the Father for what matters to you deeply. Jesus prayed until his sweat became as blood, but he died – and in some agony. At the end of the day what really matters is not that we should all get better and live happily ever after, as in some unreal fairy tale. What alone is important is that God's will may be done, and his Kingdom come, in the circumstances of *this* experience, *this* sickness, *this* action.

The question is not about bearing suffering, enduring the pain; it is about serving God in it. In other words, it is about how life may be redeemed, and (as illuminated for all time by the manner of the death of Christ on Calvary) good brought out of evil and new life emerge from the old. Life is not about fairness or unfairness. It is often unjust, claiming the good and the innocent as its victims. Life is about making certain choices: between one action and another, between generous self-giving and selfish holding back; and it is also about what we make of the harsh, unlooked-for blows that come to us all: sickness and pain, grief and old age. None of us dare judge the life of another: that is God's prerogative, and his judgement is matched by his mercy. Those who become embittered or lose their faith or take their own life in despair may have had the dice loaded against them from the start, and none of us know whether we should have survived if we had been in their place. All I would dare claim is that it is good if we learn from our own experience of suffering or bereavement, and as a result are wiser, more tolerant, above all more compassionate. There are those who are able to use their sickness, their pain, even their dying as a time for growth and a new-found trust in the God who holds us in death as in life and will not let us go. And perhaps they are not as rare as we think.

*

There was, then, the need for this experience of mine to be redeemed, to play its part in my journey inwards, which is to say, the journey into God.

I think in a strange way three things came together to enable this to begin to happen.

The first was the moment when I suddenly knew the power of the body to renew itself against all my expectations. One day, not so long ago, I suddenly knew beyond any shadow of doubt that I had turned a corner. Human beings have within them this extraordinary life-force which is of God. For us – though not, I suppose, for my beloved dog who finally gave up the hope of seeing any action in terms of walks and began to treat me as part of the furniture – this means a renewal of the creative life-giving spirit. I do not wholly understand how it can be so, but instinctively I know that my true self is none other than God within me. Father Harry Williams, writing in *Poverty, Chastity, Obedience*, has this to say:

> God is both other than I am and also the same. For God is apprehended as the source from which I continually flow, and the source cannot be separated from that which continually flows from it . . . In my deep communion with the mystery of another person and in the mystery of my own being, what I find is God.[56]

And Oliver Sacks writes of our power of recovery:

> That a return to health is possible, in patients with half a century of the profoundest illness, must fill one with a sense of amazement – that the potential for health and self can *survive*, after so much of the life and the structure of the person has been lost, and after so long and exclusive an immersion in sickness . . . One must allow the possibility of an almost limitless repertoire of functional reorganisations and accommodations of all types, from cellular, chemical and hormonal levels to the organisation of the self – the 'will to get well'. One sees again and again, not merely in the context of Parkinsonism, but in cancer, tuberculosis, neurosis – *all* the diseases – remarkable, unexpected and 'inexplicable' resolutions, at times when it seems that everything is lost. One must allow – with surprise, with delight – that such things happen. *Why* they should happen, and *what* indeed is happening, are questions which it is not yet within our power to answer; for health goes deeper than any disease.[57]

And the philosopher Nietzsche, a man unsympathetic to Christianity but who knew much about illness, waxes positively lyrical on the subject:

Gratitude pours forth continually, as if the unexpected had just happened – the gratitude of a convalescent – for convalescence was unexpected . . . One is all at once attacked by hope . . . the intoxication of convalescence after long privation and powerlessness: the rejoicing of a strength that is returning, of a reawakened faith in a tomorrow and the day after tomorrow, of a sudden sense and anticipation of a future, of impending adventures, of seas that are open again, of goals that are permitted again, believed again.[58]

When that happens, however slowly, you are renewed (resurrected in a way) and give thanks for this showing of the powerful activity of God, 'who creates (and recreates) us by his power and redeems us by his love'.[59]

The second chance for my illness to be redeemed came from a remark made to me by Doctor D. I had asked him why he thought I was so vulnerable to the virus in the first place. 'Perhaps,' he said, with a smile, 'because your inscape does not match your landscape. I use the term', he said, 'in its Jungian sense.'

My *'inscape'*: as I understand it, my inner landscape, those truths I seek to live by, speak about, hold important. My *'landscape'*: the actual bit of the world where I function, where I am heard and observed. What I wrote of earlier is an example of where they do not match: I spoke of the community's task of caring for the lonely or listening to those who are anxious; yet how often has someone said to me, 'I nearly came to see you last month but I felt I shouldn't bother you, and it's all right – things have resolved themselves'. This gap between 'inscape' and 'landscape' is true of all of us, but it is a particular temptation of the professional, the public person; and I guess it may be a particular failure of the clergy. It leads to tension and guilt, very often unacknowledged, which can leave you drained and vulnerable.

But it goes deeper than that, for it also has to do with the expectations many people have of the priest, the tension not just between the private persona and the public man, but the tension between what you see to be proper and improper expectations. By virtue of his role, a priest represents more than himself, yet he can only function if he retains his own flawed humanity. He carries the weight of many false ideas of God which are projected onto him as God's declared representative, and it is not easy to walk the razor-edge between bearing (in the most positive sense of the word) and rejecting those false expectations. This, too, can create tension, especially when times of prayer and private renewal are allowed to be crowded out of the day, and the priest relies on his own resources rather than those of God.

But perhaps it goes even deeper still. The priest knows that, though flawed, he must try to care about and be interested in the many people who call upon his time. Mostly he does. But all counsellors know that there will be a few who not only drain them very quickly but can make them angry. Yet somehow they must repress their irritation and their anger, and it rarely finds an outlet. Over the years that no doubt adds to the mismatch of 'inscape' and 'landscape'.

'Perhaps your inscape does not match your landscape.'

That was an uncomfortable truth, and I think I might have forgotten it if it were not for Sister G, a nun who came to talk to me about prayer (mine, not hers). She listened for a while, and having listened she said just one thing: 'When you pray, try to ask the question: *What is it I really want?*' A few days later I read these words of

Father Gerard Hughes and linked them to her question: 'To make a decision according to God's will is to make a decision which our deepest self really wants.'[60]

'What is it I really want?' It is a deceptively profound question. It recalls the incident when Jesus, faced with the paralytic who had lain by the pool of Bethesda for thirty-eight years, asks him: 'Do you *want* to recover?' Many don't. It is not hard to recognise the professional invalid, who escapes from the demands life would otherwise make into the cosier, restricted world of the sickbed. But there are infinite subtleties in the games we play and the ruses we adopt in our desire for sympathy and protection from the harsh reality of life, and our need to be valued and reassured. For the priest, the one who sets out to be a healer, yet knows himself to be a 'wounded healer', may not illness be a way of resisting the expectations made of him, a cry for help because he needs people to recognise his own weakness and limitations?

'What is it I really want?' *Now*, at this critical point in my life: *now*, in this situation where I am always in the presence of God? I thought until I came to the Dolomites to convalesce that the answer was simple. I wanted my health so that I could do my job at Westminster with confidence. I desperately wanted to be fully well again. I still do.

But then, on Whitsunday, I realised that was not the point. It was during Mass in the village church at Deutschnofen, a church filled with hundreds of red and white carnations to symbolise the descent of the Spirit. People of all ages filled the nave, while the non-communicating, elderly men in their dark suits sat in the gallery, along with the choir.

The latter sang a setting of the Mass accompanied by an unusual combination of cornets, trumpets and bassoons. The people were deeply attentive, the celebration done with care. Suddenly, during the prayer of Consecration, Sister G's question (to which I had given no thought for weeks) came into my mind – 'What do you really want?' – and with it a different answer. I knew that what I wanted most of all was not to be healed physically, but *to learn the lessons of my sickness*. I wanted this lost year to be redeemed, to be a valued part of my journey. Perhaps at last I was beginning to glimpse what God had been doing all this time.

To some that may sound a little too neat, especially to those who know much greater depths of bewilderment and anxiety, pain or grief. Yet in speaking of my desire that this year may be redeemed, I am not suggesting that all our lives can have a happy ending, with everything unravelled and resolved. Redemption is what Christ achieved by the manner in which he met the full force of human sin and its consequences and the manner in which he faced the anguish of Gethsemane and the desolation of the Cross. It is about reacting to what is negative and destructive in such a way as to draw good out of it. And after the Resurrection Jesus stood among them and said 'Peace be unto you'. For them it was the final proof that everything he had said about the Father's love was true; yet he still bore the marks of the nails in his hands and the spear in his side.

Jesus did not offer people perfect health and a painless death. Human minds and bodies are fragile and vulnerable. What he offers is eternal life: a new relationship with God of such a quality that nothing that may happen to us can destroy it. And it is that kind of confidence and trust in God, *come what may*, which is the true healing of the human spirit.

But it may be the way of the Cross.

So 'I greet him the days I meet him and bless when I understand'. And I knew at that moment in the Mass that I wanted to say 'yes' to whatever Westminster may bring with an openness and a conviction I previously lacked. I love Dag Hammarskjöld's prayer and often use it:

For all that has been, thanks;
To all that shall be, yes![61]

but my 'yesses' have so often been hedged around with reservations. And will be again.

I am not yet physically as well as I shall be: the lungs still ache when under pressure, the rash still glows on my chest, my muscles remain weak and don't perform as they should, I still take the pills; but I sense that my spirit is quite different, and I know at last the intoxication of convalescence.

I am realist enough to know how quickly such moments pass and to recognise that the really hard part is still to come. But we should not dismiss or minimise these child-like moments of joyful perception – or, rather, of God's grace; for not only are they glimpses of what lies in store for us when we have finally learned to put away the childish things which so dominate our lives, but they are part of the process of redemption and make all the bad times worthwhile.

Postscript

For six months I put away my manuscript: partly to see how – from the physical point of view – the story would end; partly because I returned home to a demanding, unusual summer. It was a time of packing up and preparing for Sarah's wedding in Great St Mary's on a glorious June day. A week later I was installed at Westminster, where the most fearsome hurdle was taking the long oath in Latin, and two days after that we moved into the Deanery. A fortnight later came the Royal Wedding of the Duke and Duchess of York. By the grace of God the adrenalin flowed and I was carried through a memorable and exciting day.

As summer turned to autumn, and the honeymoon period of the new job began to wane a little, and people stopped asking how I was, I realised I was stuck. Doing more, far more, than six months ago, but physically no better: feeling ill for part of each day, with increasing weakness, aching limbs, and that persistent sense of pressure in the lungs.

When I left Cambridge someone had written: 'If you get stuck ask if you can see Dr H. He is an eminent neuro-physician and should be able to help.' My new GP wrote to him and asked if he would see me as a National Health patient. He agreed. A fortnight later Alison and

I drove to Oxford. Dr H was a man who wasted no time. He asked me to describe my symptoms, then gave me a very thorough examination. Then he invited Alison to join us and explained with the greatest clarity what he thought was wrong. He picked up, as it were, all the bits of information we had been fed from time to time and made sense of them.

'At first you had something very like glandular fever, though it wasn't that, but a severe viral infection. What you have now is what some people call the post-viral fatigue syndrome, but its real name is benign Myalgic Encephalomyelitis (ME for short). It is a chronic disabling condition which can in fact follow any viral infection, and some people find it very hard to get rid of.'

He went on to explain that people may suffer some striking muscle (myalgic) fatigue, that they may get severe pain in the chest or elsewhere, and not be able to walk more than a hundred yards before feeling exhausted, together with disabling mental (encephalo) problems, such as confusion, loss of memory and lapses of concentration. The first recorded cases in Britain were in 1955 and many doctors still remain unaware of its widespread nature. (A recent radio programme about ME brought a huge demand for information, and there may be as many as a hundred thousand ME sufferers in the country.)[62]

The key abnormality would seem to be that an otherwise healthy person gets a viral infection and his or her immune system (the defence mechanism in the body) fails to make the appropriate response.

The virus is thought to 'hijack' the genetic material (DNA) [writes a doctor who has himself suffered from ME for eight years] and use it to manufacture new viral particles. The specialist white cells that normally co-

80

ordinate the body's immune response, known as T-lymphocytes, fall in number, producing a chronic immune deficiency picture similar to that seen in AIDS . . . Once the syndrome becomes established, the long-term outcome is unpredictable. Some make a virtual or total recovery – often those able to rest completely in the early stages before the diagnosis has even been made. Others seem to run a more protracted course with periods of complete remission, lasting weeks, months or even years, followed by lapses precipitated by undue stress, over-work or a new infection. The third group remains constantly unwell, but fortunately very few seem to follow progressive downhill courses.[63]

Dr H, however, was encouraging. He told me he was confident I would recover, though he warned me it might take a longish time and he prescribed some tablets which have the effect of stimulating the immune system. 'And if you are not better in six months', he said, 'let me know.' It was the most enormous relief. He added something else: a short analysis of my personality which he had perceptively observed from the nature of my answers and the description of my symptoms.

'I guess you are precise, a bit of a perfectionist, someone who is always putting pictures straight.'

'Yes,' I said, 'I'm a Virgoan.'

'I'm surprised you give any credit to that nonsense,' he replied, 'but so am I. And when people like us get ill we need to analyse every symptom; and that doesn't help.'

*

The change has been infinitely slow, noticeable over months rather than weeks. Pills keep the symptoms under control. There are still good days and bad days (though

81

more of the former) and the pattern is unpredictable. But there are long periods of each day when I feel well again, free of discomfort, and can even share the delight of e.e. cummings' poem:

i thank You God for most this amazing
day: for the leaping greenly spirits of trees
and a blue true dream of sky; and for everything
which is natural which is infinite which is yes . . .[64]

Yet I know now a little of what it feels like to live in the shadow-land with those whose lives are diminished; and in my better moments I am glad to have done so.

Westminster
Pentecost 1987

References

1. Gerard Manley Hopkins, 'The Wreck of the Deutschland', *Collected Poems* (OUP, 1967).
2. Dennis Potter, 'The Other Side of the Dark'. Unpublished talk on BBC Radio 4, 23 February 1977. Quoted by permission of the author.
3. Philip Toynbee, *Part of a Journey* (Collins 1981), entry for 15 March 1979.
4. Psalm 22:2 (Alternative Service Book, 1980).
5. Psalm 10:1 (ASB).
6. Psalm 13:2 (ASB).
7. Psalm 18:4, 6 (ASB).
8. Psalm 42:6-7 (ASB).
9. Psalm 139:2, 18 (Book of Common Prayer).
10. Psalm 139:11-12 (ASB).
11. Psalm 30:5 (ASB).
12. John Donne, 'Devotions V', *Complete Poetry and Selected Prose*, ed. John Hayward (Nonesuch Press 1978), p. 513.
13. Oliver Sacks, *Awakenings* (Duckworth 1973), pp. 194-5.
14. Ibid., p. 198.
15. Ibid., p. 234.
16. Ibid., pp. 234-5.
17. Montaigne, *Essays* 3, 13.
18. *The Healing Arts* (BBC Publications 1986), pp. 26, 37.
19. Andrew Rissik, a review in *The Times*.
20. W. H. Vanstone, *The Stature of Waiting* (Darton, Longman & Todd 1982), *passim*.

21. Richard Holloway, *Paradoxes of Christian Life and Faith* (Mowbray 1984), p. 49.
22. Jeremy Taylor (source untraced).
23. John V. Taylor, *The Go-Between God* (SCM Press 1979), p. 19.
24. Paul van Buren, *Theological Explorations* (SCM Press 1968), p. 169.
25. Philip Toynbee, op. cit., entry for 20 October 1979.
26. Ian Ramsey, address printed in *Spirituality for Today*, ed. Eric James (SCM Press 1968).
27. Monica Furlong, *Travelling In* (Hodder & Stoughton 1971), p. 45.
28. Sören Kierkegaard, *Christian Discourses*, trans. Walter Lowrie (OUP, New York, 1961), p. 322.
29. Ibid., p. 79.
30. Dennis Potter, op. cit.
31. Gerard Hughes, *God of Surprises* (Darton, Longman & Todd 1985), pp. 17–18.
32. Caryll Houselander, 'The Young Man' in *The Flowering Tree* (Sheed & Ward 1973). Quoted by permission of the publishers.
33. Romans 11:33b–34 (New English Bible).
34. John 1:18 (Jerusalem Bible).
35. Dennis Potter, op. cit.
36. Michael Ramsey, *God, Christ and the World* (SCM Press 1969), p. 37.
37. Dame Cicely Saunders, Address given in Great St Mary's, Cambridge, 31 January 1982.
38. John Austin Baker, *The Foolishness of God* (Darton, Longman & Todd 1979), p. 406.
39. Dietrich Bonhoeffer, *Letters and Papers from Prison* (SCM Press 1953), pp. 166, 164.
40. Geoffrey Preston OP, *God's Way to be Man* (Darton, Longman & Todd 1978), p. 23.
41. Julian of Norwich, *Revelations of Divine Love* (Penguin 1966), chapter 73.

42. I cannot trace the source, although the words have been attributed to Augustine by others. Professor Henry Chadwick writes to me: 'The words are a *very* free paraphrase and development of Augustine's ideas . . . no doubt he would be pleased to be credited with so noble a sentiment . . .'

43. Ephesians 5:20 (J. B. Phillips' translation).

44. 1 Thessalonians 5:18 (New English Bible).

45. Obituary for Father Christopher Bryant, *Church Times*, 14 June 1985.

46. William Law, *A Serious Call to a Devout and Holy Life* (published in 1728; Everyman edition J. M. Dent 1955), p. 197.

47. Isaiah 43:1b, 4a (Revised Standard Version).

48. Psalm 56:3 (ASB).

49. Hebrews 13:6 (NEB).

50. Job 30:16–17 (JB)

51. Psalm 139:7b (Book of Common Prayer).

52. R. S. Thomas, 'Folk Tale', in *Experimenting with an Amen* (Macmillan 1986). Quoted by permission of Macmillan, London and Basingstoke.

53. Peter de Vries, *The Blood of the Lamb* (Penguin 1969), *passim*.

54. Monica Furlong, 'Christus III', in *God's a Good Man* (Mowbray 1974). Quoted by permission of the publishers.

55. John Macmurray. Gifford Lectures (1954).

56. H. A. Williams, *Poverty, Chastity, Obedience* (Mitchell Beazley 1975), p. 111.

57. Oliver Sacks, *Awakenings*, p. 202 and note; p. 230.

58. Friedrich Nietzsche, *The Gay Science*, Preface for the 2nd edn, 1887.

59. Collect for Morning Prayer, Alternative Service Book 1980.

60. Gerard Hughes, op. cit., p. 140.

61. Dag Hammarskjöld, *Markings* (Faber & Faber 1964), p. 87.

62. The address of the M.E. Association is: P.O. Box 8, Stanford le Hope, Essex SS17 8EX.
63. Dr Charles Shepherd, article in *Vogue*, October 1986 (Copyright: Condé Nast Publications).
64. e. e. cummings, *Selected Poems 1923–1958* (Faber 1958), p. 76.